P9-CBP-755

Elderly Care

This volume provides specific examples in practice of some of the strategic principles outlined by the author in his report to the United Nations entitled *Aging: Programme Recommendations at the National Level for the Year 2001.*

Alexandre Sidorenko
Officer in Charge, United Nations Ageing Unit,
Vienna, Austria

Elderly Care
A world perspective

Edited by Ken Tout

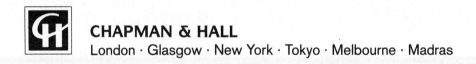

CHAPMAN & HALL

London · Glasgow · New York · Tokyo · Melbourne · Madras

Published by Chapman & Hall, 2–6 Boundary Row, London SE1 8HN

Chapman & Hall, 2–6 Boundary Row, London SE1 8HN, UK

Blackie Academic & Professional, Wester Cleddens Road, Bishopbriggs, Glasgow G64 2NZ, UK

Chapman & Hall Inc., 29 West 35th Street, New York NY10001, USA

Chapman & Hall Japan, Thomson Publishing Japan, Hirakawacho Nemoto Building, 6F, 1-7-11 Hirakawa-cho, Chiyoda-ku, Tokyo 102, Japan

Chapman & Hall Australia, Thomas Nelson Australia, 102 Dodds Street, South Melbourne, Victoria 3205, Australia

Chapman & Hall India, R. Seshadri, 32 Second Main Road, CIT East, Madras 600 035, India

Distributed in the USA and Canada by Singular Publishing Group Inc., 4284 41st Street, San Diego, California 92105

First edition 1993

© 1993 Chapman & Hall

Typeset in 10/12 Palatino by Expo Holdings, Malaysia
Printed in England by Clays Ltd, St Ives PLC

ISBN 0 412 47630 4   1 56593 141 6 (USA)

A catalogue record for this book is available from the British Library

∞ Printed on acid-free text paper, manufactured in accordance with ANSI/NISO Z 39. 48-1992 and ANSI Z 39. 48-1984 (Permanence of Paper)

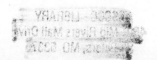

Contents

Note: Chapters marked * have been translated and/or given their final English form by the Editor.

About the contributors

Julia Tavares de Alvarez, Ambassador, is Alternate Representative of the Dominican Republic to the United Nations in New York and co-founder and President (pt) of the Banyan Fund.

Aloyzio Achutti, a geriatrician, is chairman of course studies in the Faculty of Medicine at the Universidade Federal do Rio Grande do Sul in Porto Alegre, Brazil, where his wife **Valderes Robinson Achutti**, also a geriatrician, collaborates with him.

Nana Araba Apt, Senior Lecturer at the University of Legon, Ghana, is President of the African Gerontological Society and a founding member of HelpAge Ghana.

Antony J. Bayer is a geriatrician at the University of Wales College of Medicine, Department of Geriatric Medicine in Cardiff, Wales.

Miriam Bernard is Director of the Centre for Social Gerontology in the Department of Applied Social Studies and Social Work of Keele University, UK, and was formerly with the Beth Johnson Foundation.

Vladislav V. Bezrukov is the Director of the Institute of Gerontology of the Ministry of Health of the Ukraine, in Kiev.

Mohamed Boulasri is Directeur des Affaires Sociales, Ministère de l'Artisanat et des Affaires Sociales, Kingdom of Morocco in Rabat.

Myriam Buhagiar is Coordinator of the Good Neighbours Scheme of Caritas Malta at Caritas headquarters in Floriana, Malta.

Vera V. Chaikovskaya is an associate of Dr V. V. Bezrukov at the Institute of Gerontology in Kiev, Ukraine.

Nelson W.-S. Chow is Professor and Head of the Department of Social Work and Social Administration in the University of Hong Kong.

Enid Opal Cox is Director of the Institute of Gerontology at the Graduate School of Social Work, University of Denver, Colorado, USA.

Guillermo del Pozo Veintemilla is to be Director of the newly established National Institute of Gerontology at Vilcabamba, Ecuador, and is President of Asociación Pro Defensa del Anciano de Vilcabamba.

Roberto Dieguez Dacal is Principal Specialist in Geriatrics and

Gerontology of the Dirección Nacional de Asistencia Social of the Ministry of Health, in Havana, Cuba.

J. Robert Ekongot is Projects Officer of HelpAge Kenya in Nairobi, Kenya.

Denise Eldemire is Senior Lecturer in the Department of Social and Preventive Medicine, University of the West Indies, and Joint Chair of HelpAge Jamaica in Kingston, Jamaica.

Zaida Esquivel is Directora Operativa (Operational Director) of AGECO, the Costa Rican Association of Gerontology, in San José, Costa Rica.

Eduardo Garcia Jacome with his wife **Rita Duarte** is a co-founder of Pro Vida Colombia, of which he is President, and also a co-founding Vice Chairman of HelpAge International.

Mario Garrett has been Programme Manager and Coordinator of INIA, the International Institute on Aging (United Nations) in Valletta, Malta.

István A. Gergely is a geriatrician at the Gerontology Center of the Semmelweis University of Medicine in Budapest, Hungary, and is Vice President (from July 1993) of the International Association of Gerontology.

Sharon Gordon is an educationalist and gerontologist at the Lake View Terrace Retirement Community in Altoona, Florida, USA.

Dalip L. Kohli is a former Lieutenant-Governor of Delhi and is a current Trustee and former Director of HelpAge India.

Alex Y.-H. Kwan is Principal Lecturer in the Department of Applied Social Studies at the City Polytechnic of Hong Kong.

George W. Leeson is Director of Research and Development of the DaneAge Foundation, Copenhagen, Denmark.

Kai Leichsenring is a researcher at the European Centre for Social Welfare Policy and Research in Vienna, Austria.

Linda Machin is responsible for the only Certificate course in Bereavement Counselling in the UK, at the Department of Applied Social Studies and Social Work of Keele University.

Luise Margolies of the Universidad Central de Venezuela is the Director of EDIVA (Ediciones Venezolanas de Antropología) of Caracas, Venezuela.

Sister Pacifica McKenna has worked for 50 years in the Beni region of Bolivia as teacher, nurse, therapist and latterly Director of the Hogar (Home) Sagrado Corazón in Trinidad town, Beni.

Marie Mills teaches and studies at Southampton University on 'Aspects of Dementia' and also owns and runs a residential home for 20 elderly persons in Hampshire, UK.

Kayoko Minemoto is a researcher of the Osaka Institute of Community Social Services and teaches at Sonoda-gakuen Women's Junior College, Osaka, Japan.

Meredith Minkler is Professor of the Community Health Education Program at the School of Public Health of the University of California, Berkeley, and co-founder of the Tenderloin project in San Francisco, USA.

Andrew C. Nyanguru is Director of the School of Social Work in Harare, Zimbabwe, and Visiting Lecturer, School of Social Work, University of Cape Town, South Africa.

Totaro Okada is former Professor of the School of Social Welfare, Ryukoku University, Kyoto, and Director of Osaka Institute of Community Social Services, Osaka, Japan.

J.D. Pathak is Director Emeritus of the Medical Research Centre at the Bombay Hospital, India.

Rafael Pineda Soria is Coordinator of the Plan Gerontológico of the National Institute of Social Services (INSERSO) of the Ministry of Social Affairs in Madrid, Spain.

Lyudmila A. Podust is a researcher at the Institute of Gerontology in Kiev, Ukraine.

Birgit Pruckner is a researcher at the European Centre for Social Welfare Policy and Research in Vienna, Austria.

Jan Reban is a geriatrician of Hluboka, Czechoslovakia, and has been involved recently in setting up the European Exchange Centre on Gerontology in South Bohemia.

Leopold Rosenmayr is Professor at the Institut für Soziologie, in the Sozial- und Wirtschaftswissenschaftliche Fakultät at Vienna University, Austria.

Andrew Sixsmith is Lecturer in Social Gerontology at the Institute of Human Ageing of the University of Liverpool, UK.

Jai Tout is Principal Officer for Elderly Services for the Basildon Area of Essex County Council Social Services, UK.

Catherine Tunissen is a researcher at the Instituut voor Toegepaste Sociale Wetenschappen (ITS) of Nijmegen, Netherlands.

Otto von Mering is Professor and Director of the Center for Gerontological Studies at the University of Florida, in Gainesville, Florida, USA.

S.M. Zaki, retired naval commander, is Vice-President of the Pakistan Senior Citizens Association in Karachi, Pakistan.

ABOUT THE EDITOR

Ken Tout is an Honorary Research Fellow of the Centre for Social Gerontology of Keele University, UK; First Visiting Lecturer in Transcultural Gerontology at the Center for Gerontological Studies of the University of Florida, USA; and lectures on international ageing at universities in several countries. On retirement from an appointment as International Coordinator of HelpAge International he set up his own Consultancy in International Ageing, CONSULTAGE, in 1991. He has worked on consultancies with the United Nations Ageing Unit and the World Health Organization.

For 12 years, in the 1950s and 1960s he lived and worked in South America and southern Africa, being associated with welfare and developmental work of international voluntary agencies including Oxfam and Help the Aged, with whom he also served as Press Officer at their British headquarters. He has written numerous articles on ageing in addition to the references in this book. He was founder editor of the *AGEWAYS* and *ageAction* bulletins. He has also written three acclaimed books of war memoirs and, after service in World War II, his first post-war tasks included working with elderly people in blitzed cities of the north of England.

For most of the 1980s he was also Director of Help the Aged (UK) grant aid programme in Latin America and the Caribbean and travelled extensively in the region to stimulate the setting up of local research, innovative projects, and age care organizations. With his wife Jai in 1985, at the invitation of the Belize government, he undertook a national survey on ageing and prepared a plan for a national programme on ageing.

PART ONE
Introductory

*All corresponding statistics throughout the book are from Mario Garrett's 1992 study of United Nations medium variant estimates for 1985.

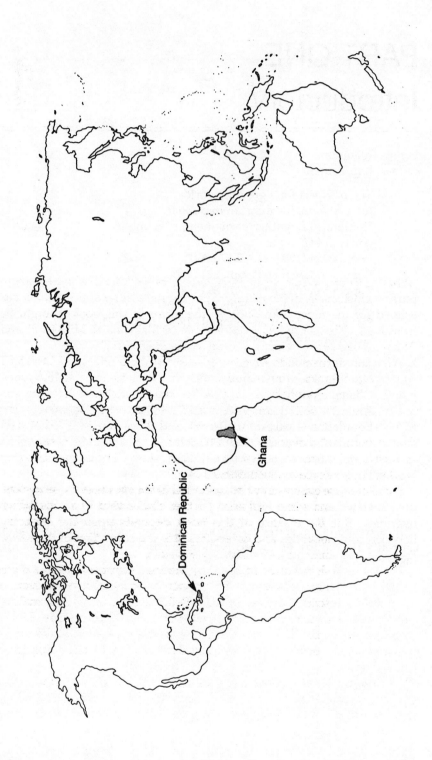

Intention

Ken Tout

'What's Hecuba to him, or he to Hecuba ?' is the kind of Shakespearean phrase which sticks in the memory. During the editing of this book it has echoed for me more than once. In the terms of this book it might be translated 'What's Minkler to McKenna, or Mckenna to Minkler ?' and 'What's Kohli to von Mering, or von Mering to Kohli ?'.

What affinity could possibly exist between the denizens of Minkler's concrete jungle and the fading cowboys of McKenna's living green jungle? What commonalities can exist between an architect planning von Mering's luxury retirement village and a volunteer builder following Kohli's suggestions and using mud and husk walls ? What few similarities must there be between Jai Tout's frail, confused Essex elders in their royal name bungalows and Nyanguru's lusty crop-cultivating workers in the outback of Zimbabwe ?

Some of those queries must be answered in the course of those writers' own reviews and some will need further elaboration in a concluding overview. But the essence of this book depends upon the interplay between commonalities and diversities. It is the conviction of the editor that each has something of value to say to each.

From the lush pastures of the von Mering retirement village there emerges the universal concept of 'affinity bonding'. From the simple adaptations described in fine detail by Kohli there results a new realization that the simplest concept is often the best. To try to provide elderly people with facilities which are uncomfortably palatial is almost as unacceptable to many of them as a standard of life which is below their fondest desires.

It will soon be recognized that the editor of this book set out with the concept of achieving 'width' rather than 'depth'. To include so many themes and projects within the print space available meant sacrificing some amount of detail and perhaps of academic profundity. But, to one who travels extensively, the world has now become so exciting with a plethora of initiatives in ageing that it was time to take a panoramic view. So the book serves as a 'sampler' or 'taster' of ideas which can be enlarged upon in other works to follow.

It is also fair to say that, after a dearth of interest in – or information about – international ageing in its fullest sense, there are now appearing studies which do examine certain aspects of ageing in more depth than in these pages. Kane *et al.* (1990), Kendig *et al.* (1992) and Kosberg (1992) are good examples of this.

This book avoids specialist geriatric issues. It also largely omits religious considerations which are of utmost importance to many very old people. It seeks to cover as wide a variety of socio-economic matters and visit as many differing cultures as possible. Some articles are brief reports of small projects recently initiated. Other articles deal with a wider and more general theme. Some writers wished to include a number of references. In other cases there were few, if any, other published accounts which might have been used as references.

Consequently a certain unevenness will be apparent in treatment, breadth of theme, amount of detail and literary style. In a number of cases, particularly from the Spanish language, the authors have provided material in their own language and kindly agreed that I should translate this into English and give it a final form. This would explain some obvious uniformity in the sections treated this way.

Chapter headings are inevitably a little arbitrary as a number of contributions overlap from one sub-theme to another. Also the discriminating reader may query the omission of references to certain subjects, programmes or countries. In defence it has to be said that, with a tight time schedule and a vast task of international communication to be undertaken, there were instances where preferred programmes were unable to make a contribution to the book and, in more than one instance, either the British postal system or some faraway offender failed to produce consecutive responses. Even the fax machine ran into a cul de sac on occasion.

In choice of a title there is always the problem of inadequacy of terms. Much of the novel thinking portrayed in these articles concerns support and provision of opportunities to act, rather than imposed care as such. The term 'care' is therefore to be understood in its widest meaning as the outcome of caring, which in turn will sometimes mean leaving the older person to his/her own resources with some risk to that individual.

Another difficulty is with the terms 'elderly', 'ageing', 'older' and so on. I have not striven for uniformity but left each author's terminology as far as possible undisturbed. However I have elsewhere pointed out (Tout, 1989) that, as in the 'Vilcabamba' and 'Potosi' factors, there are places where it is common to find persons of 90 and even 100 years of age continuing to work contentedly in an exceptional state of fitness, and mental alertness. In other places it is not uncommon to find 'burned out cases', persons who are physiologically 'aged' at the age of 40.

The term 'ageing' again raises the problem of English-English and American-English spelling. I have decided on uniformity, using the English-English, except in direct quotes or titles where 'aging' and 'centers', etc., may make their more logical appearance.

This book is not the result of an idea which sprang fully developed from the present editor's brain. It had been discussed between Richard Holloway and Wally Harbert. When it seemed useful to widen the scope from a purely British domestic or European Community treatment to take in experiences from far distant and 'newly ageing' countries, Wally (who was then my colleague at Help the Aged) considered that such a task would be more in my line than his own.

As with many works of this type, there was the near catastrophe of another change of horses in midstream. As I was almost drowning in despair I was glad to find Rosemary Morris and Catherine Walker (a Minkler pupil) piloting a lifeboat to the rescue.

I had access to, and greatly value, information from the files of the United Nations Aging Unit in Vienna, HelpAge International, the International Federation on Ageing and the International Institute on Aging in Malta.

Among the individuals who in one way or another gave me support or considerable encouragement along the way (in addition to the named contributors and references in the book) were Adelbert Evers, Christopher Beer, G.C.J. Bennett, Edit Beregi, Mario Garrett, Frank Glendenning, Mgr Victor Grech, Fr Joe Hampson, Ken Johnson, Leonie Kellaher, Charlotte Nusberg, Katrina Payne, Jim Schulz, Alexandre Sidorenko, Camillus Were and Gerard van der Zanden.

I trust this volume may introduce students to this challenging and rapidly growing field of study; inspire planners and practitioners to lateral thinking in adapting or drawing the essence from programmes described; lead other researchers and writers to essay more indepth treatment of sub-themes to which they may develop a lasting commitment; and convince national and local authorities that not only is ageing one of the potential crisis subjects of the future, but there already exist many worthy models for action in which official departments can collaborate with community groups, voluntary agencies and elders themselves, to offset the threat of catastrophe before it fully develops.

The nomination by the United Nations of the year 1994 as the 'International Year of the Family' enables the 'elderly' constituency to reiterate the dual importance of the family as an elders' support mechanism and of the grandparents as an integrated educating and motivating force of the highest importance within the family structure. The identification by the United Nations of 2001 as a target date for implementation of new strategies on ageing leaves time for effective measures to be researched, planned and achieved in every country.

The prospect for a greying world   2

(Dominican Republic)

Julia Alvarez

I believe that when it comes to the subject of ageing, we are about to live in more interesting times than the colour grey might suggest. In fact, red and black would be more to the point. What will be the colour of the ink at the bottom of society's balance sheet when ageing populations make unprecedented demands on our national resources in the coming decades? Particularly in our Third World, where still another social burden could finally strangle the crucial process of development?

The increase in the absolute numbers and percentages of older people worldwide will generate tremendous demands for new social services – including special care for the very old. This will be enough to swamp all economies, unless we begin to get ready soon.

While the ageing of populations will challenge every nation, it will most dramatically affect the poorer, Third World countries. In 1975 the Third World held three quarters of the world's people but only half those over age 60. By 2025 its share of the over-60s will have grown to three quarters. The transition to an older society there will occur more rapidly than was the case in developed nations.

Among very old people, those 80 years of age and over, who are more likely to need assistance, the true revolution will also occur in our Third World. Between 1980 and 2020, the number of octogenarians will double in the more developed regions, rising in absolute numbers from 22 to 46 million persons. However, during this period in our developing countries, the number of people in this age group will increase by a factor of five, from 12 million to 64 million persons. The majority of very old persons will be living in developing countries and most of them will be women.

In our Third World, where adequate social security systems are beyond the reach of all nations, the elderly are poor first and only secondarily aged. Viewed this way, the ageing of populations is a negative factor in the developmental process, a social debit whose size will increase. Development will have a future only if the process integrates the aged as a productive asset. Otherwise, the burden of caring for greater numbers of older people with fewer resources will drag everyone down.

Rather than raise our hands in despair, we must recognize and seize the opportunity that presents itself. If we can do this, our prospects will brighten considerably.

The elderly are a national resource of great importance. They are the repository of a lifetime of vigour, accumulated knowledge, skills and experience – a veritable living database of life. Now socially and economically marginal, they must – whenever health and vigour make it possible – be integrated into development as a human resource. We must have productive ageing. This task is 'do-able'. In fact, it is already being done. Self-help, self-managed, income generating projects for elders have been brought to fruition in many Third World countries precisely because a modest investment was made available. They involve older people in raising livestock and crops they can plant and harvest without expensive machinery. In this regard, hydroponic farming is a promising field for the future. Senior enterprises also include small businesses such as laundromats and bakeries. Modern technology, far from being a barrier to the employment of older workers, has often made it easier for them to work – in wordprocessing services, for example.

There is also a successful precedent for raising the small sums needed to jump-start micro enterprises. Bangladesh has a programme to elevate out of poverty many poor rural women who have no access to credit. Since 1976, that nation's Grameen Bank has made small, unsecured loans to almost 700 000 people in 23 000 villages. It boasts a 98% repayment rate.

Other internationally oriented institutions are already building on this success. For example, the Banyan Fund, organized in 1991 under United Nations patronage, raises capital from the private sector and other non-governmental organizations to finance projects in which older people not only become masters of their own economic fate, but also agents of economic development.

The very transcending of traditional, strictly governmental responses to social problems itself bodes well for the future. It is a vindication of people such as Ken Tout, who for years has challenged us to apply common sense problem solving and to be open to new approaches. It suggests that with flexibility, intelligence and the will to act, we can do whatever it takes to meet the challenge. It offers a prospectus for a successful adaptation to a greying world.

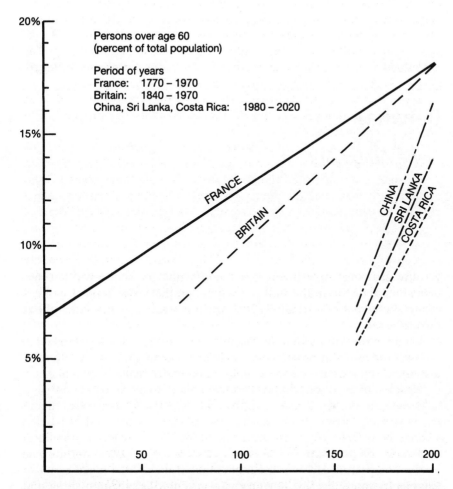

Persons over age 60
(percent of total population)

Period of years
France: 1770 – 1970
Britain: 1840 – 1970
China, Sri Lanka, Costa Rica: 1980 – 2020

FRANCE
BRITAIN
CHINA
SRI LANKA
COSTA RICA

20%
15%
10%
5%

50   100   150   200

Rapidity of ageing. Forecasts suggest that, over a 40 year period, many developing countries will undergo an increase in their elderly population (percent of total population) equivalent to that which took up to 200 years in parts of western Europe

The storm clouds are grey

3

(Ghana)

Nana Araba Apt

Worldwide forces of urbanization are affecting the social and psychological state of the individual human being, the major impact being a change in the patterns of family life. And it is frequently the elder who is most affected.

When the rural individual moves into the city he must adapt himself to a new kind of interdependence with new social groups, community institutions and organized services. In the course of that adjustment much that is good of the old traditions is rubbed off. A vacuum can ensue.

Modernization, with increased physical, educational and social mobility, is shifting people from the traditional patterns of family and clan settings. New factors of social stratification based on new forms of political leadership, modern 'up-to-date' skills, education, occupation and income have taken precedence over the more familiar ones. Traditional forms of leadership and collective responsibility are gradually diminishing and losing their former binding force which helped provide social security for older members of the extended family.

Most of the urban growth is a result of migration from rural areas. In the urban style of development the social amenities which are available in cities and large towns – although not perfect – appear to be superior to those in rural areas. Some of these advantages include tapped water supplies, sewerage, electricity, postal facilities, entertainment, educational establishments and the opportunities in business of all sorts. These logically attract mainly young people anxious to 'get ahead' in life (Apt, 1991).

For a long time the myth has prevailed, especially in Africa, that the extended family, with its structures and patterns of group solidarity and blood ties, would render virtually insignificant any problems associated with ageing. Although there is not yet sufficient empirical evidence to give conclusive proof to the contrary, observers of the African scene (where the extended family remains perhaps most entrenched) point to irreversible social and economic trends which will have detrimental effects on the remaining family structures and on ageing individuals on a wider scale if no serious efforts are made to forestall such consequences.

In my country of Ghana studies clearly indicate that ties which have bound the family from time immemorial are now rapidly loosening. As far back as 1962 the first ever survey of the aged in Ghana had some important revelations. Firstly, it showed that as many as 18% of the rural households interviewed had 'come close to having lost contact with their educated children who had migrated to the towns'. Secondly, even though financial obligations to the extended family remained very strong and on the whole such obligations were not resented, yet of all children born to the aged in the survey 'only 35% had become what their parents regarded as good providers'. Thirdly, there was an indication that 'in a ninth of all rural families and a sixth of urban ones no help had been forthcoming in old age' (Apt, 1971).

More recent studies confirm the trend (Apt, 1989), which is also apparent in most African countries. And I have listened to similar reports of more advanced family disintegration in conferences on other continents, from both industrialized and developing nations.

Annual reports of hospital welfare services since 1966 in Ghana indicate increasing concern over the number of old people aged between 60 and 90 years who have problems on being discharged from the hospital because of their relatives' reluctance to take home an aged, bedridden patient. There is further concern at reports of increasing abandonment or 'dumping' of aged persons at hospital gates.

Studies indicate that most Ghanaians, as elsewhere, are willing to take responsibility for the care of their own elders. But most young people lament the fact that economically they are unable to assist their aged relatives as adequately as they would want. These are glaring facts: it is becoming increasingly difficult for wellmeaning workers to feed and house themselves, their immediate descendants and other relatives, some of whom might be elderly.

As in many of the world's vast and still growing cities today, in Ghana's capital Accra the incidence of elderly destitution seems to be increasing. Recently the cases of elderly beggars have hit the national headlines. The Korle Wokor Society cares for more than 40 of these destitutes, providing food, clothing and other material needs including health care. The cases include many like the following:

Mr K, suffering from partial paralysis, lies on a bench in an alcove between two buildings, surrounded by his few personal belongings. No trace of any family members.

Mrs O, ejected by her son because she 'did not respect his privacy'. Sleeps on a neighbour's verandah. Has another son living in England but no contact with him.

Mr G, deserted by his wife because of his constant ill health, lived in a room with a roof half ripped off and was thus beaten with rain during the heavy rainy season.

Groups like the Korle Wokor Society, St Vincent de Paul and HelpAge Ghana are working to establish adequate welfare programmes. But many fear that the storm clouds of demographic forecasts will produce a tropical storm of destitution and it will be beyond the capacity of such groups to meet the total demand of a very rapidly greying society.

In spite of cases like those cited, many people in Africa – as, no doubt, in other regions – continue to extol the virtues and strengths of the extended family in its provisions for the welfare of elderly people. Whether the traditional extended family will be able to meet the needs of its members in the future has yet to be answered.

And change will continue to change! The question of change is still pre-eminent. The assumption is that many of this generation of elderly will have children and other relatives to watch for their well-being. But they are likely to be more secure than their children and grandchildren are likely to be when they grow old. The well-being of elderly people in a rapidly changing society has become a crucial problem which requires urgent governmental attention now – at local, national and international levels.

PART TWO
Care at home

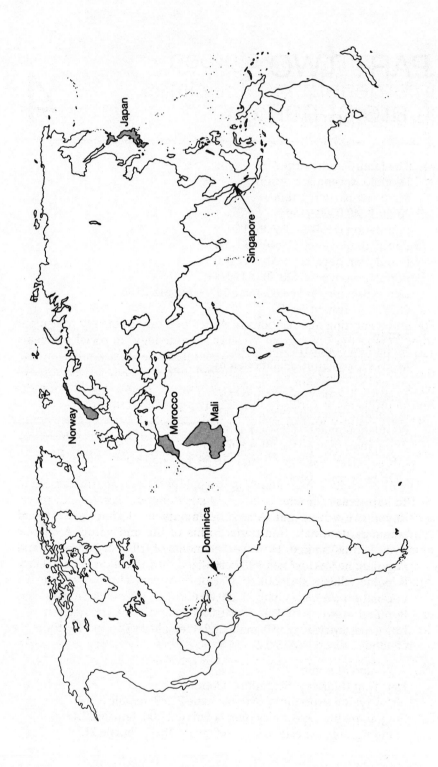

The family undisturbed – intergenerational realities in traditional Africa

4

(Mali)

Leopold Rosenmayr

For understanding age relations in Africa one cannot merely transplant some perspectives of current Western 'gerontology' to social problems and traditional cultures basically different from the West. Understanding the roots of the high evaluation of the old in the concrete setting of tribal black Africa leads us to decipher, by this paradigm, one of the most central problems of African cultures in turmoil and transition.

During a study tour in Senegal I had learned the close interrelationship between what was not solved in the rural areas and what presented itself again – maybe in a somewhat different form – as a social problem in the city.

The African cities, particularly the megalopolis type of urbanization in Africa, like areas of Dakar, Abidjan, Ouagadougou, Nairobi, etc., represent a culture where non-African elements of design, habitat and symbols may dominate traditional forms of life and value. A chaotic pluralism is thus created. However, elements of tribal organization and congregation, norms and values internalized during childhood and early youth in the villages do not and cannot disappear abruptly, neither in the first nor completely in the second immigrant generation. In the slums or populous quarters of the African megalopolis, particularly in the ethnically segregated neighbourhoods, tribal social forms continue to operate and facilitate further migration to the city by offering some sort of local protection (Attias-Donfut and Rosenmayr, 1993).

THE AUTHORITY OF OLD MEN

In Grand Yoff, one of the extended poor quarters and in some slumlike areas of Dakar, I found the authority of old men widely accepted by the local communities. Some sort of moderate gerontocracy existed in this vast, still growing, in many ways 'underdeveloped' suburban region, an area with exceptionally poor public health provisions. It was with and through old men that ameliorative projects (supported by European organizations) could be negotiated with the local inhabitants. From this lesson in suburban African gerontocracy I turned to a village study of my own in Mali (Rosenmayr, 1991).

Traditional tribal socialization as we observed and investigated it in Sonongo has the following characteristics. The relationship between the position of the old and the bringing up of the young is not a direct one with the exception of grandparents–grandchildren relations. There is no direct learning of the respect for the old, it is indirectly learned when group identification takes over as the immediate physico-emotional ties with the mother are severed, and as group ties are periodically reinforced over the life course.

In childhood socialization the relations with the grandparents are of a special character. These relations are so-called 'joking relations'. They are free of authority anxieties, are playful and close. Sexual innuendo is used openly and frequently, e.g. the grandmother praises the handsomeness and attractiveness of her grandson and affirms playfully that she will desert her husband and marry the grandson.

Early childhood after weaning is characterized by this type of free relations coupled with the security that the children's group offers. This double social partnership with grandparents on the one hand and the children's group on the other does exclude much antagonism, counter-dependency and the like. In short there is no protest phase which we could observe.

The 'Ton' organization which we found in operation in Sonongo illustrated the collective framework for the children, with peaceful community functions. Co-operative and cohesive qualities of unbroken mutual support are learned in this organization which forms a kind of help brigade and performs work which contributes to the organization of feasts. Cohesion and a spirit of fellowship and camaraderie are learned.

'Tribal closeness' is the result of these socialization processes, not individual competitiveness and achievement behaviour. As there is little room for individual competition, there is little motivation towards achievements. A system where the authority operates through groups, does not evoke a spirit of 'handling things', 'problem solving' and the like. In a way, things are expected to happen by themselves. Following the seniority principle, the system has trained people throughout centuries to wait for what the old on top will have to say and what they – the tribe members – might be ordered to do.

It seems clear that such expectations breed inertia, particularly under conditions of poverty and ecological deprivation. The sympathetic patience and readiness to adjust to unforeseen misfortune and the sometimes nerve-racking individual inertia Westerners experience in some African areas on many occasions stem from the precontractual mentality which accepts the system operation. And the system was (and in part still is) based on a seniority principle which is supported by socialization as described above. The basic message of seniority is to wait and to accept until it is your turn. But it is the system (not you) which tells you when it is your turn and how you should operate.

The social cult of the ancestors and their supporting rituals furnish a principle of social continuity and protection. The forerunners and models for behaviour – the ancestors as a spiritual group – exert a protective power. The renowned forefathers are the trusted shields to protect the living against external danger and internal (moral) misbehaviour. Ancestors may even protect against wicked witchcraft.

In Sonongo it became clear that childhood socialization well prepared the acceptance of the seniority principles, albeit in an indirect way. The group spirit to which the young children were exposed immediately after leaving their mothers facilitated the acceptance of the ancestors as a group and the agreement with the seniority principles. The 'Ton' organization and later the initiation society 'Komo' reinforce this collective mentality of and for responsibility.

Under the pressure of an admittedly often brutal and even economically dysfunctional 'modernization', individual competition and actions tied to certain time requirements (operations within time limits) become a social necessity. Then the attitudes and expectations based on the seniority principle can easily become obstacles to modernization. It is clear, therefore, that some of the most intelligent youths in the village who had come into contact with Western civilization tried to go the way of individual competition. Thereby they will, in one way or another, have to disrespect the system they originated from.

Thus we arrive at one of the important social and cultural contradictions in contemporary black African society. The contradiction is painful because rejecting the old system – for the African – also means the rejection of African identity which the young need for individual and political self-assertion. It is the collision of systems which produces generation conflict and cultural animosity. To the extent that this conflict becomes fully understood by the people themselves, new ways to achieve and practise solidarity under conditions of change will hopefully open up in black Africa.

RULES BASED ON SENIORITY

I have tried to point to clues to better our understanding of the positions of the old in the traditional tribal universe and in the transition society in subSaharan Africa. We must see this position within a universe of rules based on seniority. A stable self-sufficient and self-protecting traditional society had to 'invent' and to elaborate the most appropriate code to control the slow changes and to counteract the abrupt, often catastrophic ecological, racial or political interventions from outside. Seniority offered this code.

The 'wisdom' of the old, their power over the 'word', was the product – not the source – of their prestige. The latter was ascribed to them by the seniority principle. The knowledge and capabilities of the old men were much more the outcome of, than the cause or condition for, their power.

From my study in Sonongo I cannot speculate adequately about the future of the power of the old in Africa. Basing my opinion on this study and many other field trips, I may say, however, that the internal consistency of the elaborate mythological legitimation of the principle of seniority was and is the first integrated element to disappear. As the remnants of mythology for Africans in 'modernized' cities and villages become fragments, difficult to understand, they tend to deteriorate into folklore. Witchcraft and fortune-telling more easily and more broadly continue to remain efficient, even in urban environments. Yet modernization affects socialization (Rosenmayr, 1992).

The childhood socialization practices are crucial to the support of the seniority system, as I have tried to explain. The school, however rudimentary and inefficient it may be locally, evokes individual competition. It also stimulates the ability to contradict or at least to remain silent and definitely think differently.

The task of caring for the old becomes critical where family dramas surrounding the long term care of the elderly may be played out against impending food crisis, increasing poverty and political change.

During a field trip in Cameroon I visited several villages of the Beti tribe in the tropical forest approximately 100 miles east of Yaoundé. Some of these villages are compact settlements, other are strewn through the forest. In one of the isolated huts, made out of chopped wood, twigs and leaves, there lived an approximately 60 year old woman with a ten year old boy. Her husband had deserted her and had left for Yaoundé a decade ago, as the Catholic village chief, with whom I stayed for some days, had explained to me. Her daughter died when her boy was two or three years old. When the daughter's husband left for the city, the grandson stayed with the old woman. The child's father, living with another woman and having children with her in the city, came visiting once a year to repair the roof of the hut before the rainy season.

As the boy grew up he developed great anxieties. He felt haunted by bad spirits, ran away when somebody approached his grandmother's hut and hid in the forest for days. His grandmother feared that some day he would not return any more. On the other hand she had practically nothing to feed him on. The village charity became effective only sporadically. The children fled from the boy and would not associate with him and never took him to their families so that he would get something to eat.

They said I should keep away from the boy because he was driven by the devil. The village chief told me that everybody around was poor and therefore they could not help those two, grandmother and boy, effectively. He said he was sure that for weeks she and the boy had nothing else to eat but leaves from the trees.

I chose this story as a paradigm for the desertion of the old in the African bush. The story includes the marital problem in the phenomenon of dissolution of family ties. At a Nairobi NGO symposium on elderly women, a Kenyan woman came up with the recommendation 'to train older women to stick to their husbands, to please them and to be better wives'. The story also shows that the desertion of the old by the filial group or individual cannot easily be 'moralized' and dissolved from the powerful forces of economic survival which drive so many away from the undeveloped countryside. It does need strong 'filial piety' to support parents, grandparents or parents-in-law in the bush when young children under the costly living conditions are to be given chances of education in schools. There are parents with young children in the city who must needs 'sacrifice' their old in the bush rather than let their children run wild in the streets of the city without offering them some chance of attaining social mobility through schooling.

On some occasions conferences on ageing in Africa rather helplessly deplored 'the erosion of the traditional African family and the lack of attention being paid to the needs of the elderly people who are often left alone'. This is very true because in African societies age classes carry more power and responsibility than lineage. Under modernizing pressures, the age class structure tends to break up even more quickly than the lineage organization.

COLLAPSE OF THE PRINCIPLE

In view of the inevitable collapse of the seniority principle as the central guiding rule of African society, to me it seems that only basically new attitudes and structures will have chances to institutionalize a certain 'communion' with the old, economically as well as spiritually. It may be hoped that some of the tribal solidarity heritage of traditional Africa (which may be characterized as the 'open self' or the mythologically anchored 'twin personality') will eventually offer resources to afford ageing people a set of social and communal chances.

One basic aspect will be the extension and spreading of the much discussed primary health facilities and certain health worker capacities to the villages. The establishment of very simple village pharmacies entrusted to a basically trained, well-rooted villager would be one important point in a programme of improving health conditions for the old in the African countryside.

The socio-economic development might improve the position of the elderly in two alternative strategies. Both strategies will have to include or rather require activation. In this respect particularly old men in Africa will have to redefine their roles. Not all old men are as idle as the old Bambara lineage chiefs in Sonongo, and as a matter of fact even there we found differences among how individuals defined their roles as dignitaries. Seri Sakko, the much respected head of the Komo initiation society, instructed the young in many ways, tried to improve their knowledge of nature and if he had nothing else to do he rolled dry grass into cords. Many older Dogon men in the Bandiagara region work as weavers in their villages.

As the first strategy I see integrated projects, in which old men and women occupy a certain place and play a certain relatively well defined role within a model of economically supported and socially planned development for a community or a sub-region.

The second strategy may address itself to older people as groups. Older women may be activated and trained by women's organizations in the villages where they are non-negligible forces in some regions and in some ethnic groups of Central and East Africa.

Income generating projects for the old will have to be designed and – at least at the beginning – supported from outside. Money sometimes may prove to be less important than a certain type of knowledge or skill which will lead to marketable products which the old can sell. And such products may fail to have adequate success if the groups who produce them either do not themselves have access to the market or cannot adequately control the transmission and transportation of their products to the market.

I think that both strategies ought to be tried out and carefully evaluated. It is difficult to say generally which strategy under which condition will hold more chances for success. But it seems clear that wherever elderly are 'integrated' with projects of the total population in which all age groups benefit, families will be less likely to consider the care of the elderly relatives a burdensome task.

In general, with all reference to tradition and the necessary reliance on the traditional solidarity of the 'open self', new social models will have to be introduced. Otherwise the old traditions, helpless in the face of the new socio-economic and cultural conditions, will be despised rather than used for the flexible continuity which Africa may need now more than any other spiritual and practical value.

Family realities 5

Survey by Moroccan Ministry of Labour and Social Affairs

Mohamed Boulasri

In current debates on age care in an ageing world the question of family support for the elderly takes a central place. For developing countries there is the problem of a weakening family structure. For industrialized societies there is the question of whether the weakened family structure can be rehabilitated. But, as yet, relatively little has been said, often because of taboos, about the real quality of family care.

Morocco is a country where the tradition of care for the elderly by the extended family still holds good to a considerable extent. In peasant society it can be examined and assessed. In urban and other industrial areas the structure is already under considerable strain. So much emerges from an extensive ministry study (MAAS, 1985).

At the 1982 census 6.2% of Morocco's total population was over the age of 60. Within this statistic the percentage in urban districts was only 5.4%, but in rural areas it was 6.9%. This was already a reflection of the migration of large numbers of younger people either to the nation's large cities or out of the country altogether. The movement of younger people left an increasing percentage of elderly within the peasant society.

A massive increase in the gross numbers of elderly is forecast. Taking 1980 as the 100 index, by the year 2005 the 60 to 74 age band index is expected to reach 219; the 75 and over age band would be 211; and the index of the total population just 204. Moving on to the year 2025 those same age band indices would be 530, 406 and 298 respectively. This not only suggests a fivefold increase in the 'newly elderly' range and a

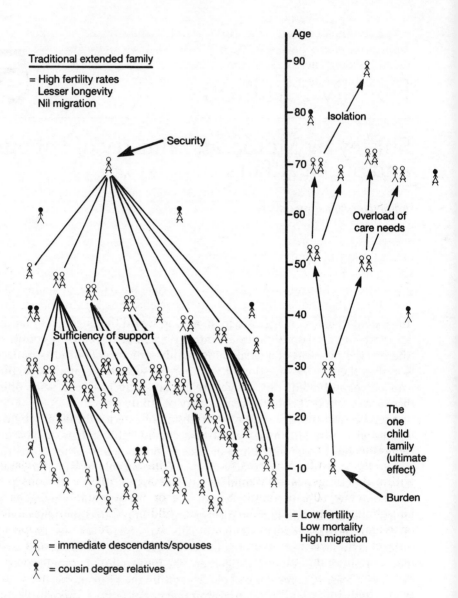

Traditional extended family

= High fertility rates
  Lesser longevity
  Nil migration

Security

Sufficiency of support

Age

Isolation

Overload of care needs

The one child family (ultimate effect)

Burden

= Low fertility
  Low mortality
  High migration

👤 = immediate descendants/spouses

👤 = cousin degree relatives

Breakdown of the family and how it affects the elderly person fourfold increase in the 'old old' bands, but a very considerable increase in all elderly compared with the increase in younger age groups.

Morocco is a country where the Islamic requirements of respect and support for elders have traditionally been strictly observed. Those ideals are still widely cherished but are under increasing pressure from various modernizing influences. One section of the government survey comments:

> Cette fréquence réduite des visites inter-familiales. . .c'est parce que la famille élargie a tendance à se réduire en raison de l'urbanisation de plus en plus rapide. (The extended family tends to be reduced because of the more and more rapid urbanization.)

Cultural considerations made difficult the researchers' task of obtaining an accurate knowledge of circumstances within families of elderly people. Language was found to be imprecise, with a gap between the formal questionnaire idiom and the evasive answers received. There was evidence of 'Islamic magnanimity' in quickly forgiving and forgetting hurt within the family. The researchers were often thought to be representatives of 'The Authorities' to whom little should be divulged. There were strong cultural concepts of the sacrosanct nature of name and ancestry so that the family's solidarity must at all costs be maintained in the public eye.

One tactic used by the researchers was to ask two or more widely spaced complementary questions which did not immediately appear to be related but which, on analysis, produced interesting results. For instance, to a direct question 71% of elderly said that they had no family problems. However, when questioned under another heading as to the need to find solutions to strife within the family, 60% of the sample had needed to find such solutions and only 10% claimed to have actually found means to resolve strife.

A pressure on families was found to be inadequate spatial provision within dwellings. The national norm was a rate of five persons per family, while 60% of families had five or more people living as a household. About 15% of elderly had no children, 32.5% of families lived on average two people to a room and 13% lived on average 2.5 people to a room. However, the average elder living within a family was in a household having three people to each room. Again, in answer to separate complementary questions, 43.5% of the elderly did not complain about those conditions when asked a direct question, but 65.5% later said that they desired better dwelling accommodation, 36% cited more space and 14% wanted 'independence' or to be on their own, or simply to have 'a place to live'.

In terms of income, many elderly persons had a mixed income (e.g., pension plus continuing work, or savings plus family aid). So, breaking down the total income picture, about 24% of elderly people's income came from retirement pensions. However, retirement pensioners were usually urban-based and linked to the public or semi-public sectors. The largest block of pensioners came from the armed forces, about 17% of all retirees. 'Administrative functionaries' came next with over 13%.

FAMILY SUPPORT

The percentage of elderly persons' income which came from personal aid was only 2.55%, added to 3.22% of 'various' (excluding pensions, wages, commerce, agriculture and property income). Forty four percent of elders received no income aid from their families. Some 36% were in regular receipt of family aid, but that aid, as indicated above, amounted only to 2.55% of elders' total incomes. Twenty five percent of those who received no family aid were in the lowest income bracket at what was then considered to be only a quarter of the adequate income figure.

In terms of family visits to elderly persons living in their own houses, the picture appeared to be more positive: 17% said they received visits weekly or even more frequently, 75% sometimes received visits and only 8% never had a family visitor. But on analysis it proved that the 75% of 'sometimes' visits related mainly to Muslim religious events, marriages or funerals, and had little aid or affection input.

Turning now to situations within the intergenerational family group, only 4% of elders interviewed gave a firm negative complaint about their family's treatment of them and 21% abstained in one way or another from a positively favourable reply. This left a considerable majority giving the positive response but often in a manner which aroused the questioners' suspicions. A more accurate picture was thought to exist in other indirect indicators and also in the many casual 'throw away' remarks made by elders outside the formalities of the questionnaire.

Among comments made by older persons about their relationships with younger family members were the following – many of them emanating from the majority who answered the formal questionnaire in a positive vein:

> We just put up with them....the youth of our day is difficult.
> My children just don't think... we simply put up with them.
> One day it is good, but other days 'No'.
> Youngsters these days are difficult.
> All those who find work abandon me.
> Each one is occupied with his own affairs.
> We have little in common.
> Since I have been retired it is seldom that they pay me a visit.
> As long as you have means, all is fine.
> Nobody bothers with me – when I had means they were all here,

but now that I have nothing nobody knows me.
The family doesn't serve for anything, it is never of help.
Get old, and people will watch out for you less, even people of your family.

An enquiry on freedom of choice produced only 45% of elderly persons who could subscribe to the statement. 'I always feel free' (to act). But again the unscheduled remarks were illuminating, such as:

I have no liberty. It is simply that my children have taken me in their charge.
An old one like me, what freedom is it possible to have?
I don't feel free because I have a family and children.
Times have changed. We have become the children of our children. We are not free any longer.
The pauper has no liberty, it all depends on your means.
You don't know anything any more about liberty when you have such problems and when you don't have enough to eat.
I am all alone. The persons I used to meet with are no longer there. And people now do not comprehend the language of other days.

FAMILY CONFLICT

On the subject of direct intergenerational conflict, as stated above, some 60% of elders had need to find solutions for situations encountered. Their 'off the cuff' comments followed similar lines:

Conflicts are obligatory...with my children who are not proud of being paupers.
I'm not happy when I have to come back home with empty hands.
One day there is a quarrel, one day none.
Lack of means slackens the ties.
The young don't take account of us.
It all depends on the day and the income.
When my children do not help me....

Desperate solutions were sometimes sought and the survey mentions significant references to the possibility of elder suicide without quantifying these. Specific remarks were:

I go off and leave them for three months or more at a time.
I go off to the country.
I leave the house and am then all right.
I pray to God to give me death to set me free.

The survey says that 'the element of comprehension has lost ground in the face of economic evolution and the progress of education'. That judgement leads on to further individual commentary:

> I am listened to when they have need of me.
> The poor one is never listened to.
> My opinion is accepted when they find it convenient.
> Each one does as he wishes, even the infants.
> Nobody consults me.
> In this house the opinion is that of the husband.
> The husband is everything in this house. (The last two comments refer to sons-in-law.)

A further enquiry covered the aspect of injury to the older person's honour, prestige or personality. This proved a difficult concept to define and convey. About 60% of elderly interviewed sensed some injury at some time. The majority cause was thought to be lack of income on the elder's part – 29% responding thus. Individual comments again reflected intergenerational attitudes:

> One has to bow one's head to the youth of this age.
> Young people today do not respect anyone.
> We have no understanding with the young ones who do not live in the same world as us.
> Respect is rare in the homes of younger people today.
> As regards my children, nobody respects me. They only respect people with means.
> Things are not like they were. Old people are no longer respected.
> Is there any young person who listens to an old person?

Younger persons revealed a 57% majority believing more or less in three common myths about ageing which were discussed, namely:

> When one ages one no longer knows what one is doing.
> Old age makes you lose your reason.
> Above 70 years of age there is nothing but complaints and illnesses.

This last myth attracted a majority of 66.5% with only about 19% categorizing it as false.

Whilst not quantified, the report does indicate a greater stability and intergenerational respect among peasant families as compared to urban groups. In many peasant families the older persons are still the land-owners with considerable skills and knowledge of low key types of agriculture, horticulture or rural crafts. Even so some 75% of rural elderly, many of them heads of household, confessed to having experienced some degree or other of loneliness because of intergenerational incompatibility.

PERCEPTIONS RAISE QUESTIONS

The survey was, of course, mainly subjective and did not use indepth objective assessment methods. It was mainly directed at the perceptions of the elderly themselves with only minor attitudinal commentary from younger generations. Thus it did not seek to allocate 'blame' for inter-generational infractions between different age groups.

The survey had the benefit of the expert guidance of two outstanding French gerontologists, Lambert and Paillat, and was led locally by a distinguished Moroccan, Professor Bentahar. It raised, or confirmed, questions sufficiently serious to justify the responsible ministry in pressing ahead with recommendations for national action, both to try to reinforce the family structure where it was still effective and to rectify erroneous attitudes which were widely evident.

Among the principal objectives propounded were to introduce social measures to delay the moment when elderly persons became a dependent charge on family or society; to aid families to assume their traditional responsibilities (as in recommendations 25 to 28 of the Vienna International Plan of Action on Aging, of 1982); to encourage rural development to reduce the exodus of youths; and to reintegrate returning migrants, especially on their retirement home from other countries.

The national plan of action would be threefold:

1. Education and awareness, analysing, explaining and changing attitudes to ageing and the elderly;
2. Short term, with focus on the abandoned, the severely handicapped and otherwise vulnerable, and to introduce experimental pilot projects with intersectoral co-operation;
3. Long term, especially in extension of health services, major construction of adequate dwellings and social protection, both financial and service delivery.

In this plan there would be two significant overall considerations:

1. The Government would have a *rôle-pilote* but would not be expected to have direct control of all means of elderly support.
2. There should be no recourse to large institutions of residence for the elderly. The emphasis should be on natural groups, with such elements as day care and night support added, to avoid institutionalization.

The priorities would appear to be to enable the older person to survive content in and through his/her own capabilities and to evolve group support either within reinforced family settings or in suitable equivalent substitutes.

To support the family   6

The 'Domiciliary Services Providing Station' in Osaka, Japan

Kayoko Minemoto and Totaro Okada

The average lifespan of the Japanese in 1991 was 75.9 years for males and 81.9 for females, the longest in the world (Ministry of Health and Welfare, 1991). Since 1950, the birthrate in Japan has declined rapidly and is now the second lowest in the world. This, in turn, has brought about a rapid increase in the ratio of elderly people to the entire population, at present about 12%. Although this is not remarkably high compared to Western countries, the ratio is expected to increase rapidly in the remaining years of this century. By the beginning of the next century, Japan will have one of the highest percentages of elderly in the world.

What is most significant now is the increase in the number of the very old aged 75 and above. The number of very old people will rise substantially until 2025 when they will constitute about 50% of all elderly people. The significance of this is that they will make the greatest demand on health and social services. Bedridden elderly totalled approximately 520 000 in 1981 and it is expected that the number will double by the year 2000. In the same year, the number of elderly suffering from mental impairment was approximately 540 000. The Government also estimated that there will be a dramatic increase in the number of elderly who suffer from mental impairment.

In Japanese families, 40.4% of the elderly still reside with their married sons and another 34.8% live with their children's spouses. There are several factors which influence the living arrangements of the elderly in Japan. First, the high percentage of the elderly living with their children can largely be ascribed to Japanese cultural attitudes regarding living arrangements. In a nationwide survey conducted in 1981, approximately

60% of those aged 60 and over indicated that 'it is good to live with children and grandchildren' (Prime Minister's Office, 1981). Second, it can be assumed that the aged reside with their children as a result of a serious housing shortage.

THE GOLD PLAN IN JAPAN (NATIONAL GOVERNMENT)

As described above, the issues confronting Japanese ageing society and the problem of caregiving for the frail elderly are becoming serious and urgent. The ratio of the bedridden elderly is much higher than Northern European countries. Therefore, the Japanese Government has begun to campaign to 'reduce the bedridden elderly to zero'.

In December 1989, the Ministry of Health and Welfare (MHW) with the co-operation of the Ministry of Finance (MOF) and Ministry of Home Affairs (MHA) developed the Gold Plan. This plan is a 'ten-year strategy to promote health care and welfare services for the elderly'. Its aim is to develop both domiciliary and institutional welfare services.

In response to circumstances, various social welfare services must be provided at home so that the elderly can live with their families and communicate with neighbours even when they need help. Thus, municipal governments have to cope with this phase and develop their own social service programmes. The development of home help, temporary stay (short-stay) and daytime services (day care), as well as the establishment of domiciliary care support centres, have been encouraged.

DOMICILIARY CARE SUPPORT CENTRES (ZAITAKU-KAIGO SHIEN CENTRES)

Domiciliary care support centres are 24-hour centres staffed by professionals at locations nearer than a municipal office, providing care for the elderly at home. This support system is modelled closely on the system of social services in northern Europe and the UK. However, the Japanese programme has been modified to account for the different cultural attitudes, special Japanese family type and views about family caregiving.

The Domiciliary Care Support Centres Programme was established in 1990. At that time there were 300 centres. By 1999, the Gold Plan will have 10 000 centres in operation. Half of the expenses for construction and operation are subsidized by the MHW. Each centre consists of a social worker or health nurse who coordinates the services and a nurse or welfare 'caretaker' (registered careworker) who provides instructions on how to care for the elderly.

The staffing and services provided are as follows:

1. Professionals (social workers or health nurses) who give advice on difficult living situations and coordinate various welfare services;
2. Nurses or welfare caretakers (registered careworkers) who instruct the families on how to take care of the frail elderly, known as 'family caregivers school' (*kazoku-kaigo kyoshitsu*);
3. Display and demonstration of aid equipment;
4. Collaboration with community welfare volunteers (*minsei-iin*).

In the past, institutions for the elderly, such as Homes for Elderly Persons (*yogo rojin home*) and Special Nursing Homes for Elderly Persons (*tokub etsu yogo rojin home*), only provided services to the elderly living in the above institutions. Currently, the operation of the welfare institutions is at a turning point. In order to keep the elderly and handicapped in their own homes, the concept of 'normalization' has become widely accepted.

Most of the domiciliary care support centres are, at present, operating in conjunction with special nursing homes in order to provide the same services to the elderly and their families and to support them in continuing to live at home. In other words, the goal is socialization and generalization of the institutions to the community. In Japan, social welfare services have been provided upon application.

DOMICILIARY SERVICES PROVIDING STATION IN OSAKA PREFECTURE (*ZAITAKU SERVICE KYOKYU STATION*)

The main purpose of the station is to provide respite for caregivers and the following services are actually available:

- home help;
- daytime service;
- temporary stay (short-stay);
- domiciliary care support centre.

These four services are put together in one home for the elderly and this comprehensive service system is called the domiciliary service providing station. Differences from the simple domiciliary care support centre are (1) the handicapped as well as the elderly can avail themselves of it, and (2) there is a director who is an expert on welfare and integrates the project to link and strengthen its four main functions. Fourteen stations have already been established in Osaka Prefecture. At least one station per city/town (43 in all) is planned to be established in the future.

LUTHER HOME

Luther Home is located in Shijo-nawate City, Osaka Prefecture. The city is relatively newly developed and is a satellite of Osaka City populated by approximately 50 000 people. Four thousand two hundred of these are over 65 years and the rate of the elderly is 8.4%. This percentage is lower than the national average, but this area is expected to catch up with the national level. Eighty elderly have been bedridden at home for more than six months. The number that live alone is 450. Shijo-nawate City used to be an agricultural district but has been urbanized recently. Nuclear families are increasing; however families with three generations, which provide a high level of mutual support to its members, still remain in the majority.

Luther Home was founded by the Lutheran Churches in 1965. Its origin was a home with moderate fees for the elderly (*keihi rojin home*). It is a voluntary organization with a special social status as a social welfare institution, which is a prerequisite for running welfare services in Japan (*shakaifukushi-houjinn*). In 1977, a 50-bed special nursing home opened, followed by a day service centre. Thus Luther Home became a comprehensive institution. This institution is non-governmental, but the expense of its operation is subsidized by the state and the municipalities.

State and municipality-regulated charges for these services are as follows:

Home help service	0 to 650 yen per hour
Temporary stay service	2000 yen per day
Daytime service	800 yen per day

The staffing of the domiciliary service providing station at Luther Home is as follows: the director is responsible for the four units; the domiciliary care support centre has a health nurse and a case worker; the home help service calls on five home helpers; the five bed temporary stay service requires a social worker, two nurses and a care worker; whilst the daytime service employs a nurse, seven care workers, a driver and a nutritionist. The staff members of the temporary stay section are working both in the station and nursing home and four care workers of the daytime service section are part-time.

Luther Home station pioneered a special transportation service for the elderly who require prescriptions from the hospital or need a check-up at a health centre.

A TYPICAL CASE IN LUTHER HOME

Yoshiko Tanaka, a 74 year old woman, lives with her eldest son (43 years old) and his wife (38 years old). Her family had been farming for several generations, but her son quit farming and now works for a company. Her relatives and kin live nearby.

In 1982, the death of Yoshiko's eldest daughter gave her a great shock and initiated her symptoms of senile dementia. Parkinson's disease was added in 1990 to aggravate the dementia. The daughter-in-law became so exhausted that she began to join the family caregiver school in Luther Home. While taking the two month course, she learned care techniques and shared her problems and distress with her classmates. A health nurse at the centre worked as a coordinator to ease her situation. Yoshiko's brothers and her second and third sons were strongly opposed to disclosing their mother's dementia to the public. They also opposed visits to a psychiatrist for diagnosis and medication. The centre encouraged them to accept social services.

Yoshiko began to join the daytime service twice a week and to utilize the temporary stay for approximately ten days a month. Taking the advice of the centre, she started to use aid equipment such as a walker (walking aid), a wheelchair and head gear and now enjoys more outdoor activities, especially taking walks.

The daughter-in-law (*yome* in Japanese) in the extended family (three-generation-household) in this community takes it for granted that she will take care of her husband's mother (the so-called *yome*'s duty), and feels guilty about enjoying herself. Professional staff try to change this feudal idea, supporting the daughter-in-law's right to freedom from this burden, but try to maintain a high quality of care for her mother-in-law also.

EVALUATION OF PROJECTS

Since the activities of the domiciliary care support centre in Osaka Prefecture have just started, we will evaluate it briefly according to what has been done in Luther Home as described above. Generally there has been a positive evaluation by the community.

- It has a family caregiver school, where caregivers can be instructed and advised on how to take care of the elderly. It supports caregivers.
- Accessibility to services has been enhanced enormously.
- The community welfare volunteers (*minsei-iin*) do outreach for the domiciliary care support centre, functioning as a liaison between the centre and the families of the elderly.
- The daytime service and the temporary stay service relieve the family.
- Bathing service is provided (a very important service for the Japanese).
- Through regular visits, home helpers and health nurses from the centre can monitor the condition of the elderly and can supply the various health and welfare services when needed.

Several characteristics of needs and conditions specific to Japanese society are recognized in the case of Luther Home. First of all, a good number of the elderly still live with their family as described. In many areas, family ties are very tight and the *yome* (daughter-in-law) is impelled by a strong sense of duty toward taking care of her parents-in-law. Also the Japanese worry a lot about how they themselves are evaluated by the neighbourhood and the society in general. The *yome* tends to give up the pursuit of her own pleasure because of her role in the family. The family caregiver school is an attempt to resolve this problem. All services at the station are aimed at caregivers' respite.

The second point is that taking a bath in a deep bathtub is one of the most popular relaxations in Japan and helps relieve fatigue. It is an essential part of the culture and its absence is felt strongly. To help the elderly bathe is much harder than to help them to take a shower, but bathing service is always desired in the elderly welfare services in Japan. One of the main purposes of joining a daytime service centre is for bathing.

The presence of community welfare volunteers, *minsei-iin*, who sustain community services, is the third characteristic. A *minsei-iin* is a volunteer who collaborates with local authorities. So far their main role has been to assess the need for public assistance and to support the families. Recently, they have begun to reach out and assess more frail elderly and their families in the community who are in need of care.

The last point is that most Japanese social welfare institutions and domiciliary service centres are managed by non-governmental organizations (special social status – *shakaifukushi houjin*), that are non-profit making but under the social welfare laws and governmental supervision.

One problem of the domiciliary care support centre project relates to medical services. Though one of the main functions of the centre is 24-hour reception, when people need help in the night it is usually a medical emergency. Because the centres do not have any doctors in the night and during holidays, the elderly person is usually taken to hospital by ambulance. The seriously ill elderly cannot therefore rely on the domiciliary care support centre in an emergency. It is argued that a 24-hour system ought to have medical staff.

At present, the domiciliary services providing station in Osaka is still a pioneer project. This practice seems to be indispensable for a normalization and supply system of social services. Therefore, it is expected to be developed extensively.

All found at home 7

Initiatives to enable elders to continue at home (Norway, Singapore, Dominica).

Ken Tout

The welcome trend in support of elderly persons in many places is towards enabling them to remain in their own homes. Where the elder lives alone or with a peer relative or friend, a substantial input of services may be necessary in cases of physical or mental deterioration. Where a younger person, usually a woman, has general care of the elder a somewhat different 'package' of support may be necessary where the enabling of the carer is called for, rather than the enabling of the care receiver.

The journal *Ageing International* featured a considerable variety of enabling programmes of this kind in its December 1989 number, among them the Norwegian examples below (*Ageing International*, 1989).

NORWAY

AMMERUDHJEMMET SERVICE CENTRE

This is found in the suburbs of the capital Oslo and is a non-governmental service. The centre itself has a nursing home facility but this is used primarily as a short-stay service. The centre is adjusted according to care receiver demand and its staff can extend or retract according to that demand. This is because the home care workers also work with the client in the nursing home.

A major feature of the home care service is that the workers, who might be regarded as basically of the home help status, are given additional training so that they can render more specialized services and thus reduce the number of workers needing to invade the person's home. This is especially of benefit to confused, shy or fearful elders.

So the home care workers, apart from their availability for common domestic tasks about the house, are in effect nurse aides as well as general problem solvers. They have knowledge of how to bring in practitioners or other consultants as required and are directly responsible for the continuum of care to the client, both in their own home and at the nursing home centre. The impact on the morale of these workers is considerable so that the programme has a staff turnover of only 15% per annum compared to 50% overall in the capital.

The supporting team of physiotherapists, occupational therapists, social workers and others is charged with going out into the community to identify and respond to problems of the elders, rather than waiting at a central point to be consulted. The major task of trained nurses is the training of the home care workers and advising them rather than intervening, unless it is absolutely necessary.

The centre itself maintains an 'open door' policy so that, as distinct from some nursing homes, relatives and friends of the old persons staying at the centre can visit and have a meal with the patient. Children are also included in the 'open door' policy as intergenerational activities are heartily encouraged.

VANG COMMUNE SERVICE

This endeavours also to support elders in their own homes in this small village in the mountains. Again the basic strategy is to have carers working both in the community and in the nursing home. This time it is the community nurse who has the particular elderly person on her round. On a day when the nurse is taking her rota duty in the nursing home her elderly care-receivers will spend the day at the nursing home, receiving all the checks and weekly treatment which may be necessary. The day's activities range from physiotherapy to meals and social exchange.

Unlike Ammerudhjemmet, the Vang scheme pairs the trained community nurse with a part-time home help from the locality. The latter is required to be primarily a companion and friend for the helper, with the domestic and other chores having secondary if still essential importance.

The wearing of an alarm device when alone at home is an obligatory element of the scheme for frailer or more confused elders. Postmen, shopkeepers and other regular community actors are officially involved to watch for danger signs at the houses of elders living alone.

The programme has become of paramount importance because of the considerable migration of younger people away from such remote rural locations, leaving many elders living alone. The rules of the system are simple and comprehensive:

- services to be provided on request, or for perceived need, without delay;
- all services to be available, if necessary, in the person's own home;
- all services, health and social, come as an integrated whole;
- no time limits are imposed on case 'packages';
- service recipients pay what they can afford for the service.

The success of the scheme is marked by the amazing statistic that, over four years, the average length of residential stay in the local nursing home was cut from 125 weeks to 45 weeks. There were consequent savings in expenditure and, with great foresight, the savings were invested in improvements to the scheme itself.

One of the principles upon which the Vang scheme hinges, with its service of part-time home help/friends, is related to a fear about use of too many fulltime workers, some of them too professional, too unionized and too locked into theoretical preconceptions or personal career objectives. This could destroy the basic personal relationships necessary to allow the elder to continuing living the most natural and normal life within his/her own home without it being turned into a kind of annexe to the nursing home.

SINGAPORE

SINGAPORE GOVERNMENT SUPPORT PROGRAMME

In response to signs of breakdown in the extended family system, the Singapore Government has put into action a programme to support family care for older people in their own home, and this has some interesting aspects (Schulz, 1991).

- Intergenerational co-residence whereby married children and their parents are allowed to apply for adjoining public authority apartments; and, what is more, their applications are awarded high priority in the allocation system.
- Income tax relief at a stated level (2500 Singapore dollars) is available to someone caring for an elderly dependant and children can also claim tax relief to the total that they have contributed into their parents' provident funds.
- School curricula have been changed to include themes which reinforce traditional family mores and which teach respect for elders and this has been further enhanced by an annual Senior Citizens week, as well as a general family life education programme.
- Practical support services to the caring family have been introduced or improved, including service visits to domicile, day care, respite opportunities and encouragement for local communities to increase their efforts to support their elders. In this campaign two main objectives

have been well publicized: to keep the elderly fit and active and able to participate in the mainstream of community life; and to ensure that the chronically ill elder shall have adequate and appropriate services and family or community support to enable him/her to continue residing at home rather than be admitted to an institution.

DOMINICA

ABANDONED ELDERLY AT HOME

The tiny island of Dominica in the West Indies may not at first appear to be a site for experiment in the home care of abandoned elderly. The tradition of family care is still strong but, like many similar communities, Dominica has suffered from massive migration of younger people seeking better economic prospects. Inevitably this migration has taken the younger people out of the island and in most cases well away from the West Indies altogether.

The old people's organization which has evolved dramatically in Dominica indicates both the need and its own priorities in its title, normally shortened to the useful acronym REACH, that is, *Reaching Elderly Abandoned Citizens Housebound*. In what some might consider to be the 'tropical paradise' of Dominica, housing is essentially simple in rural areas. There is little need for abandoned paupers to live and sleep on city streets. Poverty can be strangely and dangerously attractive out on the verdant mountain slopes under the palm trees in a thatched hut, or even in a wooden shack on the town limits.

This is where the founders of REACH found their abandoned elders, one by one (Abraham, 1989). Their conditions were described as 'deplorable'. The relevance of this term is demonstrated by the need of the homecare visitors to carry all essentials with them on early visits, including hot water for bathing (!), towels, toiletries, medication, food, clean linen and clothes. Homes were usually shacks without electricity, running water or any kind of sanitation.

Known universally as 'grans', the lonely elders, many of them bedridden or highly incapacitated, came to expect from REACH a basic daily routine, including washing or bathing, feeding, attention to clothing and disposal of slops. Many, on the first visit, had not received medical or social attention for years and suffered skin wounds and infections from bed bugs or untreated bed sores. Some were incontinent, others mentally confused.

Although these superficial physical needs are now regularly addressed, the most important factor for the 'grans' is the daily contact, many of them having no other regular visitor. REACH visitors go out with the prime objective of trust and friendship bonding. Much attention is given to spiritual support and comfort, for the local elders tend to have retained the religious faith and dependence of their strict church upbringing.

Outside the normal daily visiting service, the 'gran' is linked into wider services, including domiciliary or hospital medical attention, laundry and possibly financial sponsorship. REACH also reports back to the Government Welfare Department, for such is the pride and resilience of these elders that many of them had lived in poverty for years without asking for help from any quarter.

The Dominica Infirmary is a 90-bed non-governmental facility caring for the chronically sick, abandoned and destitute elderly. REACH has entered into a joint project with the Infirmary to build a day centre there, with services of therapy, crafts, meals, exercise and baths. The day centre caters for patients in the Infirmary, persons visited by REACH and also older people who live with their families but have to be left alone all day as the families go out to work.

Past reasons for abandonment include migration (in which case the outgoing migrant sometimes fails to find the anticipated fortune in the new country), death of younger relatives, spinsterhood and also remaining families who themselves are too poor or weak to offer support to the elder. But for the future a new problem seems to be arising; the return home after many years of a pensioner who left as a young worker.

This latter situation has been identified by the present writer as the Kingston–Kingston–Kingston (or Victoria–Victoria–Victoria) factor. The youngster brought up in Kingston, Jamaica (or Victoria, Malta), emigrates, settles in Kingston, Surrey, UK (or Victoria, Australia), works a lifetime, dreams of the old home, qualifies for a pension and finally returns home to Kingston (or Victoria). But home is no longer what it was: urbanized, industrialized, modernized, maybe polluted, evacuated by its younger members, the families permanently disintegrated, traditional culture abandoned, violent or disdainful attitudes to the hitherto respected elders, peer groups scattered or rejecting the returned migrant as being a misfit or defector from the old society.

In the Kingston–Kingston–Kingston situation the retiree is not likely, armed with an ample European retirement pension or abundant North American life savings, to prove an embarrassment to the local social security fund. However, REACH sees these returnees as yet another incre-ment, added to the elders who will survive longer because of REACH's own services, to the number of older people who will be needing some type or extent of home care in the coming years.

This foreboding of REACH must have much wider international rele-vance and underlines the need to hasten on the interchange of home care concepts to enable the elder to remain where he/she is likely to be most happy and comfortable, with all necessary support found in their own home environment.

PART THREE
Community support

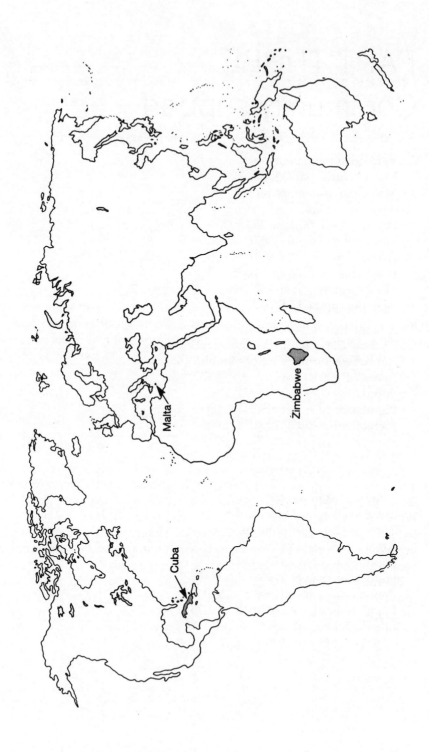

Very good neighbours!

8

The Caritas Malta Good Neighbour Scheme

Myriam Buhagiar

The Maltese Islands, Malta and Gozo, situated in the Mediterranean, have similar trends of long life expectancy to other countries in the Western world. According to the 1989 Demographic Review of these islands it has been projected that, by the year 2001, the percentage of the population over 60 years of age will be 26.2% of males and a massive 35.1% of females.

The comprehensive study conducted by the Centre for Social Research of Malta in 1982 indicated that 19% of pensioners were living alone. It also indicated that old age is a continuous process of change rather than a sudden factor of loss and decline.

As long ago as 1969 Malta was the first member state to introduce the question of an ageing population to the Agenda of the United Nations General Assembly. Malta's continued persuasion helped bring about the World Assembly on Ageing in 1982. As a result of this Caritas Malta (which had been set up in 1968) decided to introduce voluntary semi-professional services to persons in need, initiating social clubs for older persons, organized and run by volunteers in the early 1980s.

The need was recognized for the creation of a separate department of Caritas Malta for projects and programmes for the elderly, and a community social worker, Salvina Bezzina, was made responsible. As a result services are now offered to the elderly both at central and parish levels with more than 400 volunteers at work. More than 75% of these volunteers are themselves senior citizens who believe in the Caritas Malta motto of 'Helping oneself by helping other elderly persons'.

The Good Neighbour Scheme was first introduced by Caritas Malta in 1986. Dr Ken Tout, then of Help the Aged UK, and his wife, Jai Tout, were invited by Sr Salvina to take part in an eight day initial phase. The aims of this were (a) detailed planning discussions; (b) an intensive training course for the group of volunteers who would be responsible for setting up and running the programme; and (c) the creation of public awareness about problems and needs of older persons living alone, often as the result of the great emigration of younger people.

Whilst the plan envisaged today's Good Neighbour Scheme network located in 16 parishes, two localities were chosen for pilot projects: South Eastern region (Zejtun) and Inner Harbour region (Valletta, Malta's capital city). The objective of the scheme was and is to provide voluntary care, support and attention to elderly persons living alone in their own community.

The main aim of the Good Neighbour Scheme is to provide practical and regular voluntary help at the parish level to frail elderly and to persons living alone needing assistance. This service enables such individuals to remain living as securely and independently as possible in their own environment. The scheme is geared towards creating domiciliary support to prevent, wherever possible, the early settlement of the elderly in residential homes.

AN INNOVATIVE PROGRAMME

The programme has been innovative in its volunteerism in two main respects: the use of volunteers in initial discussions and in the ongoing planning and coordination at central (national) level; and the organizing of volunteer support from aspects such as transport, logistics and primary health to those volunteers who act as the actual visitors to elderly individuals' homes.

The main tasks offered by the Good Neighbour Scheme at the local level include:

- regular visits which help to offset loneliness and develop a healthy, friendly relationship, so that the volunteer will be more able to identify needs and difficulties and support can be offered on a long term basis;
- practical help for the frail elderly who find difficulties in attending to normal daily chores such as shopping, cleaning, cooking, assistance in linking into health services, transport, minor repairs and so on, which support can be arranged on a long or short term basis as required;
- check calls to provide an early warning system for those who may be at risk in their own homes. In certain cases it has been necessary to install a simple alarm system (of the door bell type) within a person's home and connected through to the next-door neighbour for emergency purposes. Even though the 'Telecare' (phone) system has

been officially introduced more recently, the demand for such a service is enormous and the resources are limited. So the Good Neighbours' voluntary emergency aid system is very practical and will be important in Malta for some time in the future.

Members of the parish Good Neighbour Scheme teams are mainly composed either of 'late adults' (50+) or young elderly, many of whom have experienced the 'living alone' situation. In this way the community group itself is giving empowerment not only on an individual basis but, in sum, on the national level. At present a total of 101 team members with 389 actual neighbours keep an eye on 672 beneficiaries of whom 268 are persons over 80 years of age and living alone.

THE NATIONAL PLANNING SYSTEM

At the central level a planning group (volunteers) works in liaison with the part-time staff community social worker to plan, organize and coordinate the scheme on a national level, always with the main aims:

1. to create national awareness about the needs and benefits of having caring and supportive neighbours in modern society;
2. to sensitize actual street neighbours to be direct or indirect helpers/carers to those living alone;
3. to coordinate the scheme from central plans to local implementation;
4. to plan, coordinate and evaluate the scheme on a national basis;
5. to provide training sessions and seminars for all 'GNS' volunteers at both central and local levels, organizing this training at local level by the teaching of flexible techniques required to initiate a scheme and then maintain it and at national level by training in the interpersonal skills of sensitive helping and watching over frail elderly persons.

THE LOCAL OPERATIONS

At the local level, parish priests have been invaluable in supporting the setting up of local schemes. First of all a limited group of motivated local persons is recruited to plan and initiate the local programme. Caritas provides a structure, system and basic training, but the actual functioning is flexible and responsive to geographical and cultural variations.

The local group undertakes a local public awareness programme, subject to the availability of resources. It then conducts a study to locate elderly persons living alone; identify the needs and difficulties of these individuals; assess the options for creating a support network; and evaluate existing offers of help by neighbours. Care is taken to avoid duplication of voluntary tasks, which could bring frustration to the volunteers and confusion to the elderly person.

As a result of the study, and recruiting more helpers as may be required, the local group is assisted by the central personnel (staff and volunteers) in setting up training sessions for the local team members who will be providing the service. After initiation of the service there is a regular evaluation and review on a six-monthly basis.

Resources are available in addition to what the Good Neighbour Scheme itself can provide immediately. In the public sector the staff and volunteers link in to official social work services. In Malta Social Security benefits are very well established and are generally sufficient for an elderly person's needs. The real problem for these persons is not in cash terms but in the existing myth of traditional caring attitudes. Like other Western countries, in Malta the cultural, religious and traditional family values are constantly changing and being overlaid by materialistic attitudes.

In 1987, Malta became the second country in the world to appoint a 'Minister' – the Parliamentary Secretary – for the Care of the Elderly. In 1988 his Secretariat introduced a home help service. This service, for which there is great demand, is normally of an hour a day or two hours twice a week. It is therefore still possible to identify needs for caring neighbours both in the daily routine and in watchfulness for emergencies. Social workers from the official programme and 'GNS' organizers work together on a mutually responsive basis to maximize their support and referrals are made both ways.

Volunteers are most useful to confused older persons in advising and helping to link up with the official home help service, the 'Telecare' system and other governmental services, as well as in claiming available cash benefits.

COMPLEMENTARY SERVICES

Caritas Malta (now 'Caritas Malta HelpAge') has initiated various other complementary projects for the benefit of elderly persons. The Good Neighbour Scheme volunteers obviously make good use of these additional options to bring support and cheer to the elders living alone. For instance, there are:

- ILAC (Independent Living Advice Centre), an initiative of Sr Salvina and Mrs Jai Tout, adapting a British model. The centre, situated in the central part of the island, has practical aids to daily living on display and these are available to the elderly. This is in line with social gerontology thinking to enable every elderly person to remain as active as possible as long as possible under their own power;

- Social clubs, now operating in 40 localities throughout Malta. The elderly people's social club opens regularly, at least once a week, to provide educational, social and spiritual indoor and outdoor activities. The clubs are run by parish volunteers. Whilst the Good Neighbour Scheme facilitates the attendance at clubs of elderly people living alone, an unfortunate trend is seen in that only between 10% and 15% of those attending such clubs are males. Elderly persons attending the clubs themselves watch for absentees, visit them and then link up with the Good Neighbour Scheme if any problem is identified;
- Minibus service is available thanks to a Help the Aged donation of a 12-seater vehicle with a tail lift. Good Neighbour Scheme group outings are a part of this service which, however, is understandably expensive as the contributions of the users do not cover all costs;
- Visiting service to residential homes is provided by another group of Caritas volunteers. So when, as sometimes happens, persons cared for by Good Neighbours eventually have to move into residential accommodation the parish Good Neighbour volunteers are able to link into the overall visiting service and maintain contact with their former neighbour.

Caritas has also published a series of booklets called *Take Care of Your Health*. The themes so far covered are *'Take Care of Your Feet'*, *'Incontinence'*, *'Dementia'*, *'Care of Your Mouth'* and *'Be Safe!'*.

The Development of the Good Neighbour Scheme continues. There is constant updating and revising of systems and methods according to changing sociocultural conditions and needs of those supported. One recent development is the greater involvement of close street neighbours – which may not have been possible in days of lesser awareness and community motivation. Two parishes have been chosen for pilot projects in greater use of immediate neighbours.

CONCLUSIONS

It does appear that public perceptions today relate more to a welfare state (delivered by government) than a welfare society (of participating individuals). This is a difficulty in the recruitment of Good Neighbours and calls for constant attention and initiatives.

Another problem relates to the role of the female in the labour market of today. This is a cause of stress within extended families. It is quite common to find 'young elderly' of 60+ and 'late adults' of 50+ taking care of parents of 80+. This causes multiple psychosocial and physical problems. The Good Neighbour Scheme does not seek to eliminate the family role of caring but to provide support and also a limited respite care service for such carers.

It has been possible by awareness programmes to obtain recognition of the principle that every neighbour in every community has a responsibility of care. Such awareness is constantly projected not only to educate community members but also to recruit more volunteers. One of the major difficulties of the programme is the continuity of finding adequate human resources.

A home that **is** its community

9

The Melfort Old People's Co-operative of Zimbabwe

Andrew C. Nyanguru

Historically, respect for the elderly was a core value in the cultures of the people living in modern Zimbabwe. Older people had a clear role to play within the rural community and the responsibility of local villages to provide for the physical and emotional security of the aged was recognized.

Kinship systems based upon consanguinal ties facilitated the absorption of the elderly within caring networks. However, the urbanization and industrialization of Zimbabwean society, with its concomitant emphasis on the nuclear family, has resulted in a loss of security and prestige for the growing population of the nation's aged.

The institutionalization of the colonial economy, however, eroded the economic position of the elderly. For those people who had been employed in mines, industry, agriculture and in domestic service, no financial security in the form of pensions was provided. They were expected to return to the rural villages when they retired. This was particularly difficult for migrant workers from neighbouring countries like Malawi, Mozambique and Zambia as they did not have rural homes and land rights in Zimbabwe. Most had lost ties with relatives in their country of origin.

As a result of the declining rural economy, the recent introduction of the Structural Adjustment Programme and the lack of an adequate social security system in Zimbabwe, many of the nation's elderly interviewed in studies were found to be destitute (Muchena, 1978; Hampson, 1982; Nyanguru and Peil, 1991). Specifically, they were without resources to pay rent or buy food, clothing and other necessities. Many respondents reported that they had no one to look after them and that they slept in the open.

It is some of these destitute African elderly people who are placed into institutions. Presently in Zimbabwe there are 71 old people's homes and 20 of these care for African destitute elderly. The homes are divided into three categories. The 'A' schemes provide sheltered accommodation in which individuals live independently in their own home but have access to a local warden in case of need. 'B' schemes provide meals, laundry service and the general care of residents. Finally, 'C' schemes are for the sick, frail and handicapped (Nyanguru, 1985).

There has been a very rapid increase in the number of homes for the African aged after independence. Sixteen homes have been established with none being established for the European and coloured communities (Nyanguru, 1990).

MELFORT: A UNIQUE CO-OPERATIVE

The aim of the establishment of Melfort Old People's Co-operative was to provide accommodation for destitute elderly, as well as to try a different method of care, where old people could live a community life each contributing according to his/her ability and receiving according to his/her needs.

PROJECT DESCRIPTION

Melfort Old People's Co-operative is a unique and innovative old people's home established in September 1979 by a group of volunteers who formed a steering committee to run the home.

In Harare, Sister Noreen saw a lot of displaced people, due to the liberation war, and among them were elderly people. She provided a midday meal for these elderly but in order to have a long term solution to their plight, the committee decided to find land on which they could live and feed themselves. They would engage in agricultural work. Land was found at Melfort, 42 kilometres from Harare. The elderly were to live as a co-operative and activity was to revolve around agriculture.

Initially there were 31 men and seven women, but the number has since increased to 42 members. Of the residents 5% are below the age of 60, 29% are between the ages of 60 and 69, 39% are between 70 and 79, whilst 26% are over 80. Seventy eight percent of the residents are male. Twenty five percent are Zimbabwean, 30% each come from Malawi and Mozambique, 10% are from Zambia, while the rest are from Angola or South Africa. Most men are bachelors whilst most women are widows. Most have no living children or relatives, and they have been migrant labourers who worked on farms, mines and in domestic service.

The co-operative is situated on some 30 acres of land of which 20 acres are arable and 14 acres are actually under cultivation. There is a small river and dam near the residential buildings where residents get household water and water for irrigation. Although there is a shopping centre about five kilometres away, there are very few human settlements in the vicinity as it is a commercial farming area. However, the home is well integrated into the community as many people visit it and the residents visit outside the home.

For accommodation, the old farm house was renovated to accom-modate about 20 men. Most of them live in a dormitory while a few share one or two bedrooms. Women have their own blocks which accommodate two or more residents. Some residents, especially women, have built traditional huts on the premises, specifically for privacy and also to enable them to prepare a special meal for themselves. There are several elderly residents who co-habit.

The material provision is what has been defined as 'resource poor' (Kosberg and Tobin, 1972). The home has no motor vehicle, TV, radio or other such facilities taken for granted by other homes. Studies I have carried out show that the residents are more satisfied with their lives than those from other homes in spite of 'resource poverty' (Nyanguru, 1987, 1990).

There is only one staff member who is called the coordinator. He sees to the day-to-day running of the home and he reports any problems to the steering committee. He lives with the residents. Among other duties, he takes those who are ill to hospital, is convenor of residents' meetings, purchases food, etc.

ACTIVE, HEALTHY CO-OPERATORS

Melfort is different from other homes in that residents are very involved in the day-to-day running of the home. The residents have a say on those who are to be admitted or expelled. Individuals make their own beds and each resident is entitled to £10 per month. They have a chance to spend their own money, compared with most homes where money is spent on behalf of residents.

Further, the residents at Melfort are involved in activities which help support the institution as well as themselves. The men have been divided into three work groups and grow such crops as maize, tomatoes, beans, etc., communally. They also raise rabbits and chickens. They share the money equally. They also have individual plots. The women also have individual plots where they grow dryland crops like groundnuts, maize and cucumbers.

Some residents have been known to buy bicycles and other quite expensive items for themselves from money earned from agricultural activities. In addition to contributing to the self-sufficiency of the home, this work increases the residents' sense of self-worth and self-fulfillment.

Social interaction among the co-operative membership is also enhanced as they participate together in productive activities. Further, the money earned in independent economic activity is used to cement friendships through the purchase of gifts, food and beer for fellow residents. Individuals also use their extra money to buy cigarettes, clothes and blankets.

Health care is an important aspect in old people's homes. When people grow old their health needs increased attention, more so than their younger counterparts. A volunteer doctor visits the home once every month. He also makes referrals for those who need specialist medical attention. A clinic/sick bay has recently been built with funds from HelpAge.

Unlike other old people's homes, Melfort buries its own dead on the farm. Residents participate in the burial of a member, either by digging the grave or any other activity. Each resident is buried according to his own cultural requirement. This information is often got from a *salwira*, who is a burial friend. One elderly man from Malawi was buried in a *vlei* (pond) near the river, because according to his culture old people are seen as children and must be buried in wet places. The *salwira* is the person who receives the dead person's clothing and belongings.

African culture emphasizes that when one dies one should be buried by relatives. In the absence of relatives, friends perform the ritual. In many homes of the African elderly, the residents are offered a pauper burial. Pauper burials mean burial by prisoners. Authorities in some homes increase the anxieties of residents by not telling residents that one of them has died. The police are called to sign the death certificate and burial order and the corpse is 'whisked away' for burial.

Some residents, even 'believers', are not given church services. This causes anxiety and because of this many African elderly say that they do not discuss death in a social gathering (Nyanguru 1987, 1990). In order to rectify this situation some elderly Africans have formed burial societies, or churches, with the hope that people will give them a proper burial.

One elderly man reported that he had joined a burial society with other members from his country. He had a friend who had joined the same burial society and agreed that, in the event of one of them dying, the other would quickly go to the burial society members to inform them about the death. These members would then intercept the corpse at the police station and take it for a decent burial. He did not want to be 'buried like a pig'. Europeans and coloureds did not show anxiety as they were usually buried by friends and relatives.

EVALUATION

There are a number of problems which have been encountered at Melfort. Participation usually assumes that someone is healthy. A number of elderly people were quite healthy when they first came to Melfort. However, for some, their health has deteriorated. This has caused a burden on the other members in terms of work load and care. There are only two 'C' schemes in the country and transfer to such schemes can be difficult. The health facilities are also not equipped for such medical conditions at Melfort.

Melfort has also had a lot of financial problems. The per capita grant of £10 per month which the Government gives is not enough to run the institution. The institution, probably because of its location, has not had the further public or private support it needs. During this drought of 1992 the elderly have not been able to grow crops which was one source of income. There has been no money to dig boreholes and there was a time when the home was threatened with closure due to lack of water.

However, Melfort Old People's Co-operative has moved away from a model of residential care facility developed during the colonial era. The social experiences of the residents in such homes are limited and the staff lead an existence quite separate from them. Inmates are subtly orientated towards a system in which they submit to an orderly routine, follow non-creative occupations and have little opportunity to exercise self-determination in their daily lives.

The situation at Melfort is different. The only staff member at the institution lives with the residents as part of the community. Daily life is not structured and co-operative members have a greater degree of self-determination in running the home. Individuals are engaged in productive activities such as animal husbandry and agriculture. These occupations are similar to the activities undertaken by the residents before their arrival. There is a sense of continuity in the lives of the residents.

Contemporary practice in the care of the aged has stressed the provision of physical facilities for the elderly. Generally, this has meant that older people have things done for them. In the process, this creates dependency. Throughout the developed world relatively expensive homes with sophisticated infrastructures are built and staffed with paid employees. However, this has not always translated into better care for the elderly living in them.

Whilst policy makers must meet the basic needs of the elderly, emphasis should not be placed exclusively on physical resources and health care. The socio-emotional needs of the elderly must not be neglected and the cultural context in which individuals have lived their lives must be respected. Melfort has even respected the sexual rights and needs of the elderly. Melfort might seem to have considered as essential components of a satisfactory residential life those defined by the Personal Social Services Council in Britain in 1975:

A respect for privacy; encouragement to independence; availability of choice; stimulation; recognition of emotional needs; opportunity to participate in organizing the pattern of life.

Residents therefore need to be involved in the day-to-day running of homes in which they live. This participation promotes the development of friendships within the facility. An added benefit, particularly in resource-poor Third World countries, is that the operating costs of such institutions are reduced as members perform the tasks that are assigned to paid employees at other facilities.

In sum, future policy in the development of residential care facilities should emphasize continuity in the conditions of life, opportunities for self-help, participation in the day-to-day running of the home and democratic decision making, all of which are needed to enhance the individual's sense of dignity and self-worth.

Alternatives to institutions

10

Various options for support of the elderly in Cuba

Roberto Dieguez Dacal

The concept of the health of man is not only related to the process of ecological adaptation but also implies an integrated vision of the reality of the individual. It must satisfy the needs and growing demands which appear over the course of life's development. The Cuban programmes to be described will therefore relate to the realization of the individual's full humanity within the existing community of whatever advanced age.

In Cuba at present the over-60s population represents 12% of the total inhabitants, but as recently as the 1960s the elderly population in Cuba did not represent a major problem as they constituted only 6% of the total at that time. In the 1960s the country could be called a demographically 'youthful' population. It was not until the 1980s that there began to be manifested the increase of this population group which enables us now to define it as a demographically 'old' population.

The greying of the population, accelerating over about 30 years, is caused by:

- a reduction in the infant mortality rate (from 27.5 per 1000 births in 1975 to 10.7 in 1990);
- a reduction in fertility rates (from 20.8 in 1975 to 17.6 in 1990);
- an improvement in the technico-scientific facilities generally.

The life-expectancy at birth has increased from 66.3 years in 1960–5 to an estimated 75.7 for 1990–5, including 73.9 for males and 77.6 for females. As will be seen our life expectancy is equal to that of a developed country, although in reality we are not that. But these demographic

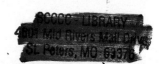

variations have made us cognizant of the fact that we have a problem to solve. Furthermore that problem will soon become larger as the various changes interact, so that it is necessary to ask ourselves:

- what will be the state of our elderly when they become 21% of the population in 2025?
- they will have more years to live but what about their quality of life?
- shall we be capable of meeting all their needs and demands?

There is what might be called 'psychosocial mortality' which can affect a person who has lost a limb or has some other serious physical impediment or mental disturbance which can mean they are suffering a living death before actual mortality. At the moment we do not know whether we can avoid such consequences or in what way we can effectively plan for massive increases in such problems.

From 1982 and the World Assembly on Ageing, there began the development of the first specialists in this field in Cuba. They were integrated into a national plan in which were included the various services which could be offered to older people through the primary, secondary and specialist services then available in Cuba.

Prominent among these options were considered self-help, family care, community support and institutional provision but a major problem affected the course of these options. Technical development led to the incorporation of the woman in work and study. In spite of the Latin American tradition of 'collective responsibility' in the care of elders, many of them now remained alone during the day. This imposed psychological strains upon what otherwise was a normal ageing process and ended by being transformed into pathological conditions related to feelings of loneliness, social isolation, depression, loss of self-esteem, predisposition to accidents, malnutrition, change in conduct (aggression, alcoholism, suicide, etc.) and poor use of leisure time.

THE 'OPEN INSTITUTION'

At the same time, and precisely because of the accelerating changes in the demographic structure of the nation, there had evolved in Havana province in 1970 a system called the 'Open Institution' (in contrast to the internment of elders in old people's homes). This had the aim of helping families who, by the nature of their work or studies, could not properly attend to their elders' needs. Medical attention, paramedical services and psychosocial rehabilitation were offered during the day and at night the elder returned to the family home. In these centres also the elders were linked into the general community by a series of varied activities.

The people called these centres *'casas de los abuelos'* (grandparents' houses) and their acceptability was such that there are now 43 such

centres in the country with a total of 3452 elders linked into the system. This system has also been incorporated in a unified structure with residential homes of the elderly since 1985, each drawing benefits from the advantages of the other.

The building plan of the grandparents' house is fairly uniform and can be a new construction or an adaptation of existing premises. Within there would generally be a reception room, a sitting room, a recreation room, administrative office, nursing and medical station, kitchen/dining hall (sometimes offering space for occupational therapy), patio or garden (for exercise, horticulture, animal husbandry or flower production), store of foodstuffs, bathrooms for the elderly and bathrooms for employees. There can be adaptations but units tend largely to mirror this model. Of the 43 current centres, two are new constructions while the rest have been adapted uniformly.

There is a standard minimum of staffing, based on five employees, namely administrator, social worker, occupational therapist, cook and general assistant. The doctor and nurse will be supplied by the Area Health Authority where the house is located. Daily attendance by the doctor is not necessary and normally he/she will visit once a week to check chronic illness cases. However, the nurse is required on an eight hours daily basis, both to ensure the hygienic and epidemiological control of the unit and to help other personnel in achieving the individual well-being of the elders.

Material resources are calculated according to needs, but it is regarded that 'tightness' of resources produces poor treatment of the elderly and therefore the supply must correspond to the structural nature of the house and to the numbers catered for. It is essential that the number of elders registered should not be less than 25 nor more than 60 at a time, for numbers outside these limits produce difficulties, especially when it is realized that these really are 'open centres' where an old person can walk in or leave at any moment he or she chooses to do so.

For organizational purposes the functions of the centres are broken down into three: administrative, attention and social. The administrator will, of course, have control of personnel matters, supplies and the maintenance of the premises.

The health service is governed by a panel from the house and the Area Health Authority and this will assure the balance of services so that all aspects of health can be offered, including prevention, health promotion and the integrated rehabilitation of both the elder and the family. There must be an accessible hospital base which can assure the house of secondary attention, seeing that primary assistance is offered directly at the house.

Social activities will be directed by the team but especially the social worker and the therapist, as well as the nurse, so that the full reintegration or retention of the elder within the local community can be achieved.

There will be recreational options (picnics, excursions, visits), table and salon games, TV, video, films and so on. Other activities will be 'socially useful' such as gardening, domestic cleaning, helping in the kitchen. There will be intergenerational exchanges, educating the new generation as to ageing, and re-educating the labour market, voluntary personnel, rebellious adolescents and so on.

As a means of autonomous government, there are councils of elders which help set up the house activities. Therapeutic working groups discuss ineffective methods. Family councils coordinate the service to elders with family considerations, thus relieving much of the administrative weight of the grandparents' house.

Who are the elders who benefit from the system of grandparents' houses? Old people with no support from children, but who are not gravely impeded by physical or mental deficiencies and older people who are left alone during the day, with similar qualification. It is obvious that admission of other old persons who are seriously affected with mental illness could upset the daily working of the house, so that other types of service have to be provided for them.

Taking into consideration normal working hours, the centres open Mondays to Fridays from 7 am to 7 pm, then Saturdays and Sundays from 7 am to midday, thus giving total respite during the day to working relatives. On Saturdays and Sundays the elders are offered only foodstuffs which they can prepare in their own homes, if they wish.

The centres have proved popular and useful. In the financial sense, to maintain an old person in their own home by use of a grandparents' house facility costs only US$3.10 daily compared to US$7.35 in residential institutions. However, with the growing population it was seen as necessary to look for other options, leading to the concept of 'spontaneous group action' of elders themselves, especially concentrating on the organization of their own exercise groups, outings, meetings and so on.

SPONTANEOUS GROUP ACTION

Circulos de abuelos (grandparents' circles) is the name chosen by the members themselves. Since their inception in 1986 the circles have grown to number 7500 groups with 162 000 elderly members. They organize sessions of physical exercise in parks, public squares and beaches, as well as more ambitious outings and cultural events. All the families are integrated into these events with the elders as leaders. At the same time the circle serves as a focus for contact with official services and each circle has its own mandatory link with a family doctor and his/her team.

The cost of the circle system is minimal but the system is supported in one way or another by all the official agencies which form part of the

Committees for Attention to the Elders, including the Ministries of Health, Internal Commerce, Culture and Education, the State Committees of Labour and Social Security, and of Finance, the National Institute of Sport and Recreation, as well as local industries.

A year later still, in coordination with the State Committee of Labour and Social Security, there was created, as a pilot programme, the project 'Attention to the Elder Living Alone at Home'. This has now been extended to the entire country. In this system meals are offered with various choices, such as to eat in communal dining rooms or to have the meals delivered at home; laundering and dyeing services are available at a nominal charge and domestic cleaning can be offered free of charge where needed.

These services are provided by two types of carers, paid staff or unpaid volunteers, among whom will be numbered both older people who are fit and alert and also single mothers. In this programme there are incorporated 6780 elderly for meals, 3210 for laundry and 2248 for domestic cleaning.

The Attention to the Elder Living Alone at Home is optional and the elder can apply for it if he/she wishes. It is recognized that many older people are very unwilling to accept into their own home some unknown person from outside. In the case of such inhibitions workers discuss the matter sensitively with the old person until a mutual agreement is reached and when satisfaction with the service can be guaranteed.

EVALUATION RECOMMENDATIONS

It is important to point out that all the options of services for elders are evaluated by a Municipal and Provincial Commission of Evaluation, made up of geriatricians, psychologists, social workers and psychogeriatricians who also ensure that the most appropriate option is available to each elder.

A considerable number of recommendations have emerged from the experiences of planning, initiating and maintaining the various options, and it can be said that these systems have the following advantages:

- attention to the greatest possible number of elders who often seek admission to an institution when this is not appropriate;
- solutions to family and community problems both in rural and urban zones;
- reintegration of elders into family and society, whilst maintaining their biosocial well-being;
- elimination of expensive architectural models – as in the case of building more institutions – and utilization of adaptable premises;
- savings in human and material resources in services;

- direct service to elders who still have abilities and capacity and can still be useful within the community;
- maintenance of family links, important for future years, when the family tends more and more to lack preoccupation with the elder;
- greater sensitivity within the family nucleus as to the elder, facilitating an increase in the numbers able to return to the family;
- creation of more responsibilities and increase in self-esteem of the elders involved in self-governing activities;
- maximizing the use of leisure time;
- more voluntary help with community activities of a socially benevolent nature;
- education of the new generations, helping them also to learn about their own ageing so as to arrive at retirement in a good physical condition;
- adequate maintenance of health, improvement of chronic illnesses and reduction of accident risk factors.

It is relevant to ask what problems may present themselves in implementing these types of service. The following should be taken into account.

- Calculation of the numbers of elderly and the location of the grandparents' house. As it is an open institution, if free time activities are not properly planned the elder will tend to leave the centre, coming back only for meals and for special social events.
- The adapted house must have all facilities appropriate to the numbers of elders, so a previous 'census' of elders in the local population is necessary.
- It is necessary in rural areas to adapt the programme and work at the acceptance by the elders of this type of congregated service which may be seen as an affront by some rural people.
- The house should cater for elders with ease of access to the site, for the involvement of transport imposes very heavy additional financial burdens.
- The resources must be total and the service continuous, otherwise the house of the elders becomes a mere store of some good things.
- The services which are offered are for the elder and not for the benefit of those who work with the elder.
- The family must always maintain its overall responsibility for its own elder, with a direct interrelationship with the centre.
- The control of the domiciliary services must be exhaustive and must remunerate with appropriate means of stimulus both paid employees and volunteers.
- The elders receiving domiciliary services must be convinced of their benefits, but never obligated to receive them.

- In the domiciliary system of service to the elder living alone in their own house, there is no benefit in trying to alter the style and standard of life of the elder in a drastic way, but progressively – and not merely to the taste of the carers – to work in ways which the elder prefers.
- The circles of grandparents are self-governing and should only be attended by professional teams in case of need and in keeping with the demands formulated by the members, thus avoiding organizational problems.

In conclusion, we recognize that not all the ideas described above can be useful everywhere, given the multiple variations of political systems and social strategies throughout the world in relation to services to the elderly. Nevertheless, in accordance with its socio-economic potential, each country can select what is interesting from these types of service and apply them fairly easily and urgently.

The only objective of all these concepts is to give sensitive consideration to the new and future Era of the Elder, which in former days was a mirage but already is approaching reality.

PART FOUR
Elders' empowerment

---

11 Empowerment: concept and demonstration
   Enid Opal Cox (USA)
   USA: federal republic
   Area: 9 372 614 sq km
   Population (1990 est.): 249 235 000
   Population over 60 (1950): 18 498 000
   Population over 60 (1990): 42 032 000
   Population over 60 (2050): 78 983 000
   Life expectancy at age 60: male 21.66, female 30.55
   GDP per capita: US$18 338

12 Power to the residents
   Catherine Tunissen (Netherlands)
   Netherlands: parliamentary monarchy
   Area: 41 548 sq km
   Population (1990 est.): 14 752 000
   Population over 60 (1950): 1 159 000
   Population over 60 (1990): 2 580 000
   Population over 60 (2050): 4 721 000
   Life expectancy at age 60: male 20.43, female 30.28
   GDP per capita: US$15 170

13 To security through community
   Meredith Minkler (USA)
   USA: as above

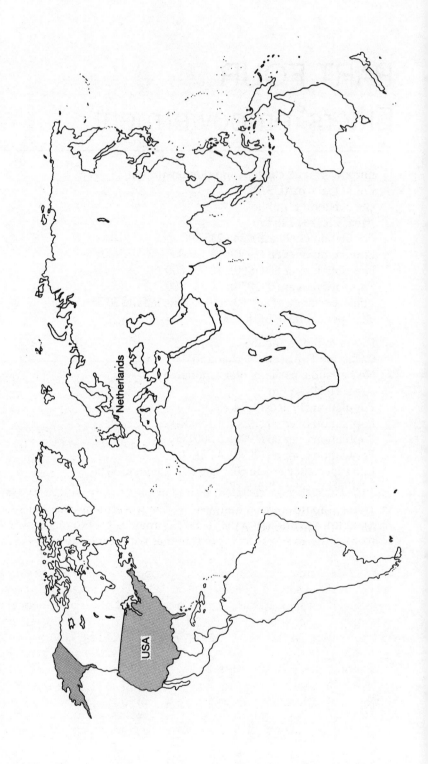

Empowerment: concept and demonstration

11

University of Denver Institute of Gerontology Empowerment Programme

Enid Opal Cox

The University of Denver Institute of Gerontology serves as a focal point of research (including social service demonstration projects), training and community service within the University of Denver. One of the key programmes of the Institute is its focus on the development of empowerment oriented services for the elderly and their families. The social work faculty at the University of Denver School of Social Work has articulated a model of empowerment oriented practice with the elderly, and the Institute has initiated a number of projects within the Denver metropolitan area which demonstrate empowerment oriented practice approaches. Additionally, the Institute provides training to agency staff to enable them to assess their programmes with respect to empowerment orientation.

There is increasing attention for the concept of 'empowerment' as it relates to social service strategies in the USA. The empowerment practice movement has appeared in response to a number of concerns about social services provision and in response to changing political, social and economic conditions in the USA. Social problems including lack of resources available to the poor, inadequate and costly health care resources and breakdown of community mediating structures (Berger and Neuhaus, 1977) are among the issues associated with the need to increase the empowerment outcomes in social services. Traditional social services have been criticized for their tendency to have a helper–helpee characteristic which focuses on the weakness or problems of clients, thus enhancing or increasing dependency. In this process the strengths and potential of clients for active involvement in the solution of problems are often neglected.

Empowerment oriented interventions have been defined for the purpose of the work at the Institute as service interventions that engage elderly clients and/or their families in:

1. the acquisition of knowledge and skills for late life survival;
2. self-help and social support activities with others sharing similar problems;
3. participation in collective/social action aimed at the improvement of their environment.

Our approach is similar to Gutierrez (1990) who defines empowerment as a process of increasing personal, interpersonal or political power so that individuals can take action to improve their life circumstances. The concept of empowerment has also been used as a principle to guide social work practice and as an outcome goal (Parsons, 1991). Empowerment oriented practice also relies heavily on an understanding of the personal, interpersonal and political aspects of problems/issues. Consequently, the problem solving process includes a consciousness raising process as a key activity.

While empowerment oriented practice can be incorporated into all methods of intervention the use of small groups has been found to be a very effective method (Cox, 1988, 1991). Gutierrez (1990) summarizes the work of a number of authors concerned with the psychological changes important to moving individuals from a sense of helplessness to action as follows: increasing self-efficacy, developing group consciousness, reducing self-blame and assuming personal responsibility for change. Small groups provide an excellent format for individuals to understand the common nature of their problems, learn about the political aspects of their problems and thus reduce the self-blame that may have contributed to their sense of helplessness.

The demonstration projects of the Institute of Gerontology are based on an empowerment oriented philosophy and incorporate at least some aspects of the empowerment oriented practice model. The following is a brief description of two of these practice demonstration projects. Each received funding specifically to demonstrate a service intervention that could later be incorporated into programmes of ongoing social service agencies.

PROJECT A: LOW INCOME ELDERLY MENTAL HEALTH PROJECT

The Institute received funds from the national Institute of Mental Health through the Colorado State Division of Mental Health to conduct a three year senior model project. The project was designed to provide an empowerment oriented group intervention for elderly residents of single room occupancy hotels (SROs). Residents of these hotels were often poor, in poor health, participants in substance abuse (especially alcohol), isolated and many had experienced identified serious and persistent mental health problems. This project was initiated in an attempt to improve the mental status of project participants. Staff consisted of second year Masters students of social work. Supervision was provided by Institute staff who have had many years of experience in gerontological social work practice.

Project methodology consisted of the implementation of empowerment oriented small groups in six sites. Workers had to spend several weeks in these facilities getting acquainted and developing a trust-based relationship with the residents in order to recruit individuals to participate in the project.

Empowerment group activities included the basic focuses of all empowerment oriented groups: education, self-help, social support and social action. Members participated in a consciousness raising process which increased their understanding of personal, interpersonal and political/economic aspects of their problems. Over 50 elderly individuals participated in these groups. Group size ranged from eight to 12 participants.

An educational curriculum was developed by project staff which included topics such as: physical, social, psychological and political aspects of ageing; health care and social service delivery systems (what is available, how to access them, issues related to the effectiveness of these services); city, state and national governments (functions, how these systems work, how to impact these systems); tenants' rights; crime prevention strategies; nutrition information; common medical information concerning prominent diseases of the ageing; legal and financial issues; and a number of other knowledge areas related to late life survival. Skills areas included advocacy, communication skills (especially how to communicate with professionals), ways to develop personal support networks, conflict resolution, negotiation skills and others suggested by the group members. Knowledgeable speakers, short audio cassette tapes and video tapes were used.

The groups were actively involved in curriculum development, identifying topics, searching for resources and presenting ideas. Many of the strategies for advocacy and/or communication came from group members. For example, one group decided that it was more effective to go in two-person teams to visit medical doctors and other professionals. This provided support to the patient as they asked professionals for information, clarification and documented events. Some members also helped to develop curriculum materials by asking experts to answer questions of interest to the group using a tape recorder so these conversations could be shared with the group. Participation of group members in an ongoing process of mutual problem solving and consciousness raising was a far more powerful aspect of the intervention than the acquisition of any specific knowledge or skill.

The group also changed from focus on the personal aspects of problems (i.e. fears, beliefs, strategies for coping with addictions, feelings of powerlessness) to focus on interpersonal dimensions of issues (relationships, communications problems, identifying common problems and concerns, mutual support activities) and political aspects of these problems (analysing the relationship of personal problems to the political situation/economy; learning advocacy and social action skills and taking various forms of action aimed at changing organizations or legislation). For example, two groups became heavily involved in advocating against the city's attempts to close their hotels due to a redevelopment effort. Any one group session could address feelings of powerlessness and anger related to the proposed evacuation, planning for presentations to city council, discussion of one member's own fears of a return to drinking as a response to the stress, setting up systems to provide interpersonal support to members of the group and other residents of the hotel, or other problems, or simply focus on one issue.

PROJECT EVALUATION

The qualitative data collected by workers and available from participant feedback were very positive with respect to intervention outcomes. Group members reported less use of hospitals for physical or mental health purposes. A number of participants demonstrated long periods of sobriety. No loss of life was experienced by group members during the move from hotels into apartments or into the new site (owners of one hotel purchased a new facility and moved the residents to the new site to avoid closing). These groups had considerable impact on negotiating the site change and on selecting apartments that allowed the group to remain intact. All of the groups involved in the projects became the core of resource and action activities in their hotel or apartment facilities. Group members reached out to other residents to share information they had, to advocate for others and to provide other forms of help and assistance.

PROJECT B: PART 1 AND PART 2 – SENIOR-TO-SENIOR MEDIATION AND CONFLICT MANAGEMENT PROJECTS

The Institute received funds from the United Way (a local community social service fundraising organization) to train 50 elderly persons to become volunteer mediators (Part 1) and to develop a six hour conflict management training module for use with elderly residents of nursing homes and senior high-rises (Part 2). Need for this project was based on community studies indicating that elderly citizens reported numerous conflict situations with families, service agencies, neighbours and landlords that affected their quality of life.

The elderly participants in Part 1 of this project came from a wide range of backgrounds (retired professionals, homemakers, homeless) and diverse ethnic/racial backgrounds. Most were active volunteers in senior service or children's service agencies of related civic programmes and planned to use their new knowledge and skills in their ongoing volunteer settings.

PART 1 – SENIOR-TO-SENIOR MEDIATION PROJECT

This project was set up to train seniors as volunteer mediators and provides volunteer mediation service to elders in Denver County. Intensive training was provided during the first 11 weeks of the project. This was followed by ongoing monthly case consultation and selected topic presentation for the remainder of the grant period. A strong emphasis of case-based learning was very well received. Participants helped to generate case material from their own conflict experiences.

Approximately 30 of the trainees were able to utilize mediation skills directly in their ongoing volunteer work. Approximately 15 volunteered to provide volunteer mediation to seniors in the city and county of Denver under direct supervision of the Institute of Gerontology. The types of disputes addressed were very diverse, including, for example, disputes in senior housing facilities regarding violation of privacy, abuse by staff members and safety issues; family disputes regarding financial issues and caregiving issues; landlord/tenant disputes; disputes with health and social service providers; disputes with other city and country government agencies; disputes regarding nursing home care; and a variety of neighbourhood disputes.

Project evaluation

Project evaluation data included feedback from participants, community service agencies in which project participants served as volunteers and from elderly who received the services of volunteer mediators. The response was extremely positive.

Project participants reported great satisfaction with the training, a high degree of usefulness of the content with respect to problem solving in their own lives as well as in their volunteer efforts to assist others. Agencies reported that the new skills had increased the effectiveness of their volunteers and in many cases led to conflict management training for other staff members. Elderly who received assistance from project participants reported very high satisfaction with the service. Even in cases where no resolution was achieved for the dispute, ratings of service satisfaction were very high. Clients were accepting of assistance from peers and felt that they could negotiate issues for themselves after participation in a negotiation process.

It is important to note that most issues were resolved by negotiation, advocacy, increased communication and mutual agreement without proceeding through all the steps of the formal mediation process.

PART 2 – TEACHING CONFLICT MANAGEMENT SKILLS TO FRAIL ELDERLY

Twelve senior mediators, trained through Part 1 of the project, worked with Institute staff to develop a conflict management curriculum for elderly persons who lived in high-rise senior facilities and in nursing homes. The goal of this project was to increase the ability of residents to solve disputes and to address their issues and concerns regarding care or other issues affecting their lives in their living situations. Problems that were identified as common to participants included: abusive staff, lack of prompt care, violation of privacy and other residents' rights, roommate disputes regarding noise, privacy, private property, safety issues in facilities, etc.

Development of the curriculum and trial sessions took almost four months. Group size averaged ten to 12 participants. Over 30 facilities were involved. The content found to be most useful for resolution of personal conflicts included: understanding one's own style of conflict resolution; alternative styles of conflict resolution; communication skills (such as the use of 'I' messages); advocacy techniques; understanding organizations; understanding professional value systems and roles. Case examples were a very useful tool, as was role playing, in assisting participants to increase their problem solving skills.

Project evaluation

Project evaluation consisted of observations from the trainers, staff of facilities and resident participants. Responses regarding the usefulness of content were solicited after each session. After the completion of the project, 30 participants were interviewed regarding the usefulness of the programme in their daily activities. All respondents reported improved communications between themselves and staff members, family members and/or roommates and neighbours in the facilities. Several reported that they felt that their communication skills had improved and that they had resolved conflicts that they would have allowed to go unresolved without the training.

Staff in the facilities were interviewed regarding changes they had observed in participants' behaviour. They reported that many of the resident participants were more assertive with respect to their needs and more effective in their communications and that some ongoing conflicts had been resolved as a result of the programme. Overall, the programme demonstrated that conflict resolution skills can be taught to frail elderly and that this process can have an empowering affect.

OTHER PROGRAMME INITIATIVES

The empowerment programme has included a number of other project initiatives that seek to incorporate empowerment oriented principles, strategies and goals into the programmes of community agencies. Elderly volunteers have been trained as peer counsellors, self-help efforts have been started in a number of high-rise facilities, residents' rights oriented programmes established in nursing home facilities and we are researching and developing care receiver interventions and service credits projects.

Care receiver interventions include: helping elders to psychologically cope with various degrees of dependency, develop knowledge to increase their capacity for self-care and the fullest possible participation in their care, the service systems that provide this care and other environmental issues affecting their lives.

Service credits projects are being developed in many parts of the country. These projects organise systems that will allow elderly volunteers to accumulate volunteer credits in return for their donated time that can be applied to pay for services they may need themselves at a later date.

OVERALL PROJECT EVALUATION

Institute staff have worked with a wide range of individuals and projects, providing training and programme consultation, in addition to directly implementing a variety of projects which demonstrate replicable empowerment oriented interventions.

Overall these concepts and efforts have been well received. The greatest barriers to expansion of the empowerment programme have been:

1. convincing some more traditional practitioners that frail elderly can benefit from empowerment oriented approaches;
2. locating programmes and staff who are able to consider innovations during a time of devastating cutbacks in social services and increasing limitation of health care benefits available to most elderly;

3. generating resources to demonstrate and sustain new methods even though they are successful.

Regardless of the difficulty experienced in expansion of empowerment oriented concepts into programming in this area, the promise of this approach is high. The increasing numbers of elderly dictate the integration and fullest participation of older Americans in their self-care and in contribution to society during their late years.

While the Institute's focus has been strongly directed on the frail elderly, empowerment oriented strategies to address the needs of more healthy elders are also indicated. Employment, housing, income and issues related to spirituality and meaningful late life roles must also be addressed using the principles of empowerment.

Power to the residents

12

Residents' Councils in Homes for the Elderly in The Netherlands

Catherine Tunissen

Residential homes (or old people's homes) in The Netherlands provide accommodation and care to elderly people who are no longer able to run an independent household. Out of a total population of around 15 million, almost 2 million are over 65 and some 7% of this age group live in a residential home. Admission to a home is not open to all elderly people, but based on an assessment of the need for care, which is made by a local intake committee.

As yet, there is no legislation at national level on the empowerment of elderly people living in residential homes. Although various proposals for Acts of Parliament have been made over the years, nationwide legislation has been postponed several times. A new Act, which covers the rights of patients and residents in different types of care institutions, is expected to be passed in 1993. At present, regulations with respect to the rights of residents in old people's homes to information and participation in decision making are set by the 12 provincial authorities, who also effectively control (among other things) the number of homes, their size and funding. These regulations vary widely from province to province and although several provinces have so far concluded evaluations of the progress being made in empowering the residents of old people's homes, it is not possible to present a nationwide view of the current situation.

THE GELDERLAND STUDY

In this chapter, I will present some first results of a study in which I was involved in the province of Gelderland. In 1991, Gelderland had 230 000 inhabitants aged 65 or over, of which some 14 560 lived in residential homes. This study was carried out in 1992 on behalf of the provincial authorities by the Institute for Applied Social Studies. It consisted of a written survey, to which 138 homes (= 75%) responded, and eight in-depth case studies. As the final report of the study has not yet been published, I will limit the scope of this chapter to the information collected on the position of residents' councils.

Residential homes are usually run as hierarchical organizations, in which a managing director makes the more important day-to-day decisions and an external board of directors develops long term policy. Participation of residents in decision making is ensured through residents' councils. The province of Gelderland changed its regulations (the so-called *Verordening*) in 1987 and in doing so incorporated far-reaching revisions in an attempt to improve the involvement of residents in decision making and developing the policies of the homes they live in.

In the *Verordening*, conditions and procedures for decision making are spelled out in detail. In many policy areas, the management of a home is required to consult both the residents' council and the employees' works council and needs their approval or advice before implementing major decisions. Each home is also required to establish a complaints committee or a separate procedure for dealing with grievances.

Another important change in the new regulations required the homes to amend the provisions in their articles of association in order to allow representatives chosen by residents and employees seats on each governing board of directors. Meetings held by the board of directors are supposed to be open (i.e. accessible to residents) and their minutes should be made public. Although the majority of homes have since revised their articles of association and over 80% now have residents or representatives of residents on their board of directors, a small number of homes are not (yet) willing to make these changes.

RESIDENTS' COUNCILS: BASIC STATISTICS

Practically all the homes in Gelderland have a residents' council. Three quarters of these councils were actually established long before the current regulations became effective. Most councils are fairly active and meet (on average) once every six weeks or so. Their activities include discussing new developments, putting forward ideas and proposals on how to deal with large and small problems, welcoming new residents, visiting residents who are ill, helping to organize entertainment, outings and other leisure activities.

Nine out of ten residents' councils are affiliated with the LOBB, a national association which actively stimulates the empowerment of residents and, among other things, sets up guidelines, gives advice and organizes regional meetings for the councils to exchange ideas and talk about anything from changes in national and provincial policies on the elderly to the day-to-day affairs of living in a home.

The size of a residents' council varies from one to nine members; most have five or six. Considering that the majority of residents are female, the proportion of men in the councils is far higher than would be expected. It is not always easy to find new members for the residents' council and ensuring continuity can pose serious problems. After all, the average age of people living in a residential home in Gelderland is 84. Frailer residents are often not willing or (physically or mentally) able to cope with the work involved, so extra support is essential. If at all possible, proper elections are held: vacancies are announced to all residents, who can then propose new candidates. The candidates with most votes are then appointed for a period of two or four years. A different method involves a more active search for new members, where council members – or the management – request likely candidates to join the council. Most councils rely on a combination of these procedures to find new members.

Just under half the councils (45%) consist of residents only. The other 55% have 'external' members also, e.g. people living in sheltered housing but not in the residential home itself, relatives of residents, volunteers or people with special expertise recruited from unions or pressure groups for the elderly.

SUPPORT AND COMMUNICATIONS

All the residents' councils in our survey receive assistance of some sort or another. Such assistance generally involves support with organizing their meetings, drawing up the agenda and the minutes, arranging transport to regional LOBB meetings, etc. One in three councils makes use of the services of a specially appointed assistant (usually a volunteer, sometimes a member of staff), who helps out when necessary but does not have the right to vote.

The general managers of the homes appear to be key figures in stimulating the councils' activities. Quite a lot of councils like to have the general manger 'at hand' during their meetings and depend on him or her to solve complaints, to answer any questions and to provide information or explanations on complicated policy matters. And although most councils meet with the board of directors once or twice a year and quite a few have direct resprensentation, contacts with the board are much more limited.

Various channels of communication are used by residents' councils to inform their fellow residents of what is going on: casual conversations (87%), notice boards (86%), publication of minutes in the home's magazine (79%), allowing non-members to attend meetings (65%), intercom system (40%), separate mailbox or suggestions box (33%). Even so, many councils find it difficult to encourage their fellow residents to participate actively.

The following inventory shows which subjects were considered most important in consultations between general managers and residents' councils:

- construction works (new buildings or renovation);
- financial situation and developments (investments, annual accounts, budgets, cuts in expenditure, fees);
- staffing policy, workloads, etc.;
- quality of care, care policy, welfare and quality of life;
- nourishment (choice anlkh;y;y;d quality of menus);
- organization of recreation and leisure activities;
- reorganizations, mergers, co-operation with other institutions.

Ideally, in decisions on such issues the views of the residents' council are heard and taken into account.

ACHIEVING REAL POWER

It is important to keep in mind that the current generation of residents are in a vulnerable position. They sometimes lack the background and experience to tackle complex issues, or may want to avoid a confrontation. Some councils therefore tend to concentrate entirely on the more trivial day-to-day problems. On the other hand, managements do not always make the effort to translate abstract policy concepts into terms the council members can understand and deal with. Some councils complain that they do not always receive vital information on time, or are even kept out of important decisions altogether. And in matters such as funding and major construction works, the province itself has the final word.

Providing an adequate structure for participation in itself is not enough. So although the first steps towards empowerment have been taken, there is still a long way to go.

To security through community

13

The Tenderloin Senior Organizing Project, San Francisco, USA

Meredith Minkler

More than 8000 elderly men and women live in deteriorating hotels and apartments in the high crime Tenderloin district of San Francisco, California. Typically providing neither cooking facilities nor private bathrooms, the 'single room occupancy' hotels in which most of the residents live constitute the bottom rung of the housing ladder in the USA. For the low income elderly in such environments, poor health, social isolation and powerlessness are often intimately connected.

A multiplicity of health problems are common among the Tenderloin's elderly residents, including high rates of alcoholism, depression, suicide, tuberculosis and undernutrition. For many residents, social isolation and social marginality lie at the base of many of the health problems experienced. Many Tenderloin elders have lost touch with family and friends. For others, limitations in physical mobility and/or fear of going out of doors in an area where elders are easy prey for criminals leave them confined to their rooms much of the time. It was toward the end of addressing some of these interrelated problems that the Tenderloin Senior Organizing Project (TSOP) described below came into being.

THE PROGRAMME: INITIAL PHASES

Originally known as the Tenderloin Senior Outreach Project, TSOP was established in the late 1970s with the dual goals of:

1. improving physical and mental health by reducing social isolation and providing relevant health education;

2. facilitating through dialogue and participation a process through which residents were encouraged to work together in identifying common problems and seeking solutions to these shared problems and concerns.

Student volunteers from the School of Public Health, University of California at Berkeley, began in a single Tenderloin hotel, offering blood pressure screening and bringing coffee and refreshments as a means of encouraging resident interaction. With the help of these inducements, an informal discussion group was formed which met weekly and included a core of 12 residents and two outside facilitators. As levels of trust and rapport increased, members began to share personal concerns regarding such issues as fear of crime, loneliness, rent increases and their own sense of powerlessness.

Student facilitators used a combination of organizing and education approaches to help foster group solidarity and social action organizing. A Freirian problem posing process, based on Paulo Freire's 'education for critical consciousness', was used to help residents engage in dialogue about shared problems and their causes and to generate potential action plans. Similarly, community organizer Saul Alinsky's admonitions to create dissatisfaction with the status quo, channel frustration into concrete action and help people identify specific, winnable issues were among the organizing precepts followed.

Finally, and drawing on social support theory stressing the importance of social interaction opportunities *per se*, the student facilitators attempted to create a group atmosphere conducive to meeting the social needs of residents as well as the more political and task oriented concerns of some group members.

As the first hotel group evolved into an established entity, seven additional groups were organized in other Tenderloin hotels. As in the first hotel, a variety of educational and organizational strategies were employed by the student facilitators and a delicate balance was sought between meeting the political/task oriented and the more strictly social needs of different residents.

Among the early issues confronted by several of the elderly hotel groups was the problem of undernutrition and particularly lack of access to fresh fruit and vegetables. Following much discussion of alternative approaches, the residents of three hotels contracted with a local food advisory service and began operating their own hotel based 'mini markets' one morning per week. In a fourth hotel, residents began running a modest co-operative weekly breakfast programme, thereby qualifying their hotel for participation in a food bank where large quantities of food could be purchased in bulk at reduced prices. Still other residents worked with TSOP staff to produce a 'no-cook cookbook' of inexpensive and nutritious recipes. Later published by the San Francisco Department of Public Health, the cookbook has been distributed free of charge to hundreds of residents of the Tenderloin and close to 1000 copies have been sold outside the community to bring in additional money for the project.

Activities like these have been important in making tangible changes (e.g. improved food access) but more significantly in contributing to resident feelings of control, competence and collective ability to bring about change. Moreover, these early accomplishments gave residents the self-confidence needed to confront more difficult challenges in the future.

THE PROGRAMME: DEVELOPMENT TRENDS

Although each hotel group developed and retained over time its own unique character, several common trends among the groups were evident. In each hotel group, for example, decreased reliance on outside facilitators was observed over time, with broader resident participation in discussions and decision making.

Greater concern for residents throughout one's hotel was also increasingly witnessed among TSOP members and was well demonstrated in the aftermath of San Francisco's October 1989 earthquake. A 75 year old TSOP member in one hotel that had to be evacuated thus was able to tell the desk clerk which of the 110 residents would need special medical attention or help getting down the stairs.

In another hotel, a TSOP member commented that while, before joining TSOP, she knew only two fellow residents, she now knew all of the tenants and felt a common bond as they weathered the aftermath of the quake together.

Another trend observed in the groups, and one critical to TSOP's evolution, was the realization among residents of the need for looking beyond hotel boundaries and working with residents of other hotels and community groups on shared problems. TSOP residents in several hotels thus identified crime and safety as their key area of concern and formed an inter-hotel coalition to begin work on this problem. The coalition in turn started the Safehouse Project, recruiting 48 neighbourhood businesses and agencies to serve as places of refuge, demarcated by colourful posters, where residents could go for help in time of emergency. Coalition members also convinced the Mayor to increase the number of police patrol officers in the neighbourhood and through this and other measures helped effect a dramatic reduction in crime, including an 18% reduction in the first 12 months after the Project's inception.

Two other outcomes of TSOP's organizing around the crime issue are worthy of note. First, having experienced success in increasing their own sense of safety and well-being, the TSOP elderly began turning their attention to the safety needs of other vulnerable groups. Recently, for example, the elderly had their Safehouse materials translated into Cambodian and Vietnamese and arranged for articles about the project to appear in the Asian language pages of the community newspaper. Armed with these materials, they were able to recruit several Asian merchants in the neighbourhood to open Safehouses. More than 80 Safehouses now operate throughout the Tenderloin and the programme has received considerable publicity locally and nationally for its efforts.

Of even greater importance, however, is the fact that some of the original founders of the Safehouse Project have continued to meet and in doing so to look critically at the need for going beyond a narrow 'crime prevention' approach such as Safehouse. Their involvement, albeit sporadic, in areas such as advocacy for the homeless, job training for the unemployed, subsidized housing and their concern with broader national policies that impact dramatically on life in this and other inner city neighbourhoods indeed reflects an increasing appreciation of the need for working toward broader social change.

THE PROGRAMME: LEADERSHIP SKILLS

TSOP has also engaged in significant leadership training, stressing one-on-one and small group activities through which residents work on improving interpersonal skills, learning to facilitate meetings and discovering ways of working through (or against) bureaucracies to bring about change. Early approaches to leadership training included a day-long leadership conference attended by 80 residents and three 'media workshops' in which TSOP members met with journalists and reporters who helped them practise articulating their concerns to the press.

Of greatest importance, however, has been ongoing individual and small group leadership training, including the extensive use of role plays prior to confrontations with landlords, meetings with city officials, etc., through which members can practise responding to alternative hypothetical scenarios. Such exercises, and the selection and preparation of back-up leaders on any given issue (to provide for continuity should the primary leader be ill on the day of a planned action), are among the strategies that have enabled TSOP to develop a strong leadership cadre from among its membership.

More advanced leadership training has also been undertaken in recent years, with several TSOP members attending intensive national leadership training programmes covering such topics as issue selection, values and critical reflection and negotiation processes.

As Tenderloin residents have increased both their leadership skills and their self-confidence, they have taken increasing control of the project, with TSOP's fulltime organizer and its student volunteers playing a less visible role, serving primarily as resource persons and 'sounding boards' for residents' ideas and strategy discussions. TSOP's mission has also been clarified over the years, with the organization gradually shedding its direct service projects in order to focus more exclusively on community organizing and advocacy within a broad social justice framework.

In keeping with this transition, the key mechanism of action within the project has changed over time from health educator facilitated support groups to resident run tenant associations. Currently TSOP related tenant organizations operate in eight Tenderloin hotels, with a total of 800 residents. Some 250 residents are regularly involved in tenant organizing activities with 30–50 of these playing key leadership roles in the project. Several additional hotels have also requested TSOP's help in organizing tenants' associations and plans are underway for their inclusion in the future.

EVALUATION AND REPLICATION

Attempts to measure TSOP's effectiveness in improving the physical and mental health of residents through reducing social isolation have proved difficult. While baseline data were collected on 200 TSOP members and controls, most residents were reluctant to participate in this and subsequent data gathering attempts for a variety of reasons, including distrust of researchers, a dislike of questionnaires and the extremely high value placed on privacy in this population group.

While effort evaluations have been conducted measuring, for example, changes in the number of support group participants and mini market patrons over time, such evaluative efforts fail to capture the qualitative dimension of the project or the real effects which these activities may have on health and quality of life outcomes.

Projects like TSOP appear more amenable to evaluation through participatory research studies which residents themselves help to design and implement. Such evaluative attempts, moreover, must examine not only individual and project specific outcomes but also changes in the larger community (e.g. reductions in crime and improvements in neighbourhood quality of life) which may be in part a consequence of the project.

In the latter regard, a significant drop in the neighbourhood's crime rate in the first two years of the project's anti-crime organizing led both police and local residents to give TSOP much of the credit for this important victory. Although the crime rate increased again in the mid-1980s, due largely to the crack cocaine epidemic, TSOP's continued anti-crime efforts contributed, according to the Mayor, to a growing sense of neighbourhood solidarity, which has itself been an important crime deterrent.

The Tenderloin Senior Organizing Project has not been without its problems. Some hotel groups have never evolved to the stage of doing real community organizing and resource limitations have left some important project activities unfunded and underdeveloped.

As a private non-profit organization with no Government or other regular funding, TSOP also faces the problem of having to raise its $100 000 annual budget largely from local foundations and individual donors. Although foundations provide about 80% of TSOP's budget, the preference of such organizations for funding specific programmes rather than core operating expenses has made this type of fundraising increasingly difficult. As TSOP has shifted to a pure community organizing project, it has found its desired outcomes (e.g. community empowerment and leadership development) less attractive to most traditional foundations than such tangible 'deliverables' as hotel based mini markets and health promotion resource centres. Moreover, even progressive foundations that have understood and applauded TSOP's new directions tend to avoid refunding the same project, so that new sources of income must be generated. Staff time, that might ideally go into helping organize new hotels, thus must be split between such work and the fundraising and related tasks necessary to keep the organization viable.

Despite these problems, however, hundreds of low income residents have been involved with TSOP support groups, tenant organizations and other activities over time and more than 300 student volunteers have gained valuable skills and insights through their work with the project. Finally, TSOP remains an effective and highly visible community based organization of and by low income elders and their neighbours and in this regard it plays an important role locally and as a model for other communities.

Attempts to replicate the project have indeed taken place both in the USA and beyond its borders. In New York City, for example, the TSOP approach has been used in organizing a community of schizophrenic war veterans and in Vancouver, Canada, it has been adapted for application in a low income elderly community. To facilitate such efforts, TSOP has produced a replication manual, describing each phase of programme development, as well as strategies and approaches that worked or failed and the essentials of community organization practice. Through such sharing, it is hoped that this model can assist elders and their advocates in other parts of the world in empowering both individual elders and the communities in which they live.

PART FIVE
Elder participation

14 Most elderly, most active
   Nelson W.-S. Chow (China)
   China: Communist republic
   Area: 9 596 961 sq km
   Population (1990 est.): 1 135 496 000
   Population over 60 (1950): 41 572 000
   Population over 60 (1990): 101 167 000
   Population over 60 (2050): 289 397 000
   Life expectancy at age 60: male 17.31, female 21.56
   GDP per capita: US$320

15 Incentives to activity
   Alex Y.-H. Kwan (Hong Kong)
   Hong Kong: British Crown colony (to 1997)
   Area: 1067 sq km
   Population (1990 est.): 5 841 000
   Population over 60 (1950): 75 000
   Population over 60 (1990): 749 000
   Population over 60 (2050): 2 001 000
   Life expectancy at age 60: male 20.90, female 27.50
   GDP per capita: US$9600

16 Senior citizens unite
   S.M. Zaki (Pakistan)
   Pakistan: federal Islamic republic
   Area: 803 943 sq km
   Population (1990 est.): 122 666 000
   Population over 60 (1950): 3 251 000
   Population over 60 (1990): 5 422 000
   Population over 60 (2050): 21 263 000
   Life expectancy at age 60: male 17.01, female 17.41
   GDP per capita: US$370

17 Their own counsel
   Ken Tout (Mexico, Australia, Argentina)
   Mexico: life expectancy over 60: male 20.37, female 23.74
   Australia: life expectancy over 60: male 20.83, female 29.32
   Argentina: life expectancy over 60: male 18.26, female 24.00

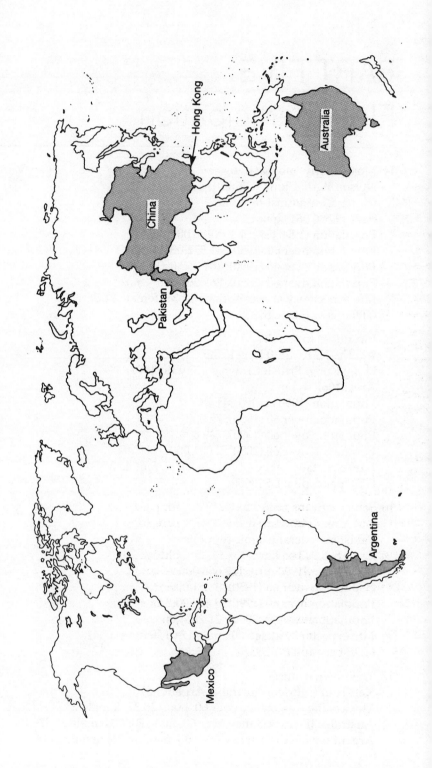

Most elderly, most active

14

Active roles for the elderly in China

Nelson W.-S. Chow

POPULATION AGEING IN CHINA

As the country with the largest number of people in the world, ageing issues in China have long attracted the interest of social researchers and planners. Although China has in the past been rather erratic in its population policies, stressing at one time the benefits to be reaped from a large population but reversing it since the end of the 1970s and restricting each family to one child, it has all along showed a keen interest in the well-being of its elderly population.

In 1982, China participated for the first time in an international conference on ageing by sending a delegation to attend the World Assembly on Ageing held in Vienna. Subsequently a National Committee on Ageing was set up in Beijing to be responsible for the promotion and coordination of educational, health and welfare activities for the elderly. Under the slogan of 'Active Participation by the Elderly,' the Ministry of Civil Affairs, which is in charge of social welfare in China, has also been organizing various projects and programmes to encourage the elderly to be active members of the community (Davis-Friedmann, 1991).

According to the fourth national population census conducted in 1990, the total population of China stood at 1.16 billion. Among them, 97.25 million were aged 60 and above, accounting for 8.57% of the total population. It is projected that this percentage will increase from 8.75 in 1991 to 14.12 in 2015 and 27.43 in 2050. If one counts those aged 65 and above, the percentage will increase from 5.65 in 1991 to 8.84 in 2015 and 20.43 in 2050. No doubt, the population in China at present is still very young, but with the enforcement of the 'one child per family' policy, it is envisaged that the proportion of the elderly will rapidly increase and the

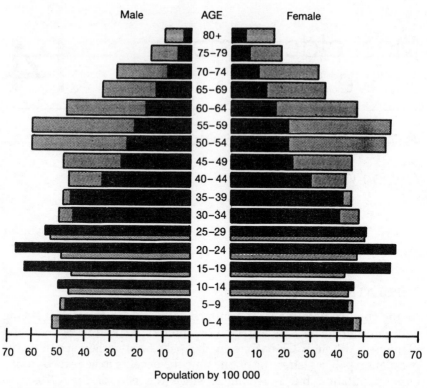

Extreme case of ageing population exacerbated by 'one child family' policy – note massive 'new elderly' group of 50–59 age bands

International Institute on Ageing (United Nations, Malta) age composition projections for China (1990 – dark, 2025 – light) (from Garrett, 1992)

population as a whole will soon become a mature one. Furthermore, the distribution of the elderly population in China is extremely uneven; while some provinces in the north west may have a small percentage of aged persons in their populations, some cities, like Shanghai, Tianjin and Guangzhou, usually have more than 10% aged 60 and above. For example, the percentage of the elderly in the total population in Shanghai as revealed by the 1990 census stood at 13.96%, which is even higher than the corresponding figure in Hong Kong.

As a result of the uneven distribution of the elderly population in China, state programmes provided for them vary greatly between provinces and from city to city. In brief, old age pensions are available to most of the retired workers living in the cities where community facilities, such as cultural and recreational centres, are also provided by the residents' committees organized in each district of the city. Provisions for the elderly in the rural areas are much inferior as retirement is theoretically non-existent in the villages and the support of the elderly falls mainly on the family. In both the cities and the villages, the role of the civil affairs bureaux is confined mainly to helping the indigent elderly and organising the residents' and the village committees to provide assistance for the elderly.

However, it is worth pointing out that though the state in China has been concerned about the increasing demand of the elderly for care and support, it sees the ageing population as both a liability and an asset. It is a liability because more public and community resources must be allocated for their support. But, as a developing country, the Chinese Government also believes that a lot could be contributed by the elderly themselves as an asset towards the betterment of society. Hence, apart from increasing the provision of services for the elderly, a number of measures have been taken by the Chinese Government to enhance the participation of the elderly in both their families and society (Chow, 1991).

MEASURES ENHANCING THE INVOLVEMENT OF THE ELDERLY

The programmes which have been introduced in various parts of China to enhance the involvement and participation of the elderly generally possess the following characteristics:

1. Usually only guidelines are issued by the responsible Government ministries or departments with the actual implementation left to the discretion of the various work units or residents' and village committees.
2. The planning of the projects must take into consideration the actual social and economic conditions of the districts concerned.
3. The moral and cultural worth of the projects is regarded as being as important as, if not more important than, their economic value.
4. The implementation of the projects must rely on the efforts of the masses and not merely the contribution of the professionals.

The following are some of the projects which have been organized so far:

- Consultative Services: In 1983, the State Economic Commission issued a directive allowing state and collective enterprises to employ retired workers as advisors and consultants. The city of Tianjin had even once organized a team of retired professionals to draw up a comprehensive plan for the redevelopment of the city.

  Obviously, some enterprises have viewed this directive with misgivings as it would imply continued control by the retired cadres, but some have welcomed this as it provides a means for the experienced retired workers to continue their contribution, though in a different capacity. However, this measure benefits only retired workers with special skills.

- Social Service by the Elderly: This programme is most commonly practised in large cities of China where the elderly are engaged in various community service projects. The services rendered by the elderly include assistance to other frail elderly, traffic patrol duties and acting as arbitrators in civil conflicts.

  It was reported in some of the large cities in China, like Beijing and Shanghai, that the involvement of the elderly in community services came up to as much as 20 to 30% of the aged population. The elderly who are participating in these community services are often doing it voluntarily but sometimes pressure may come from the residents' committees and work units to which they belong.

- Educational Involvement: Since illiteracy is still a major problem in China, educated retired workers have been involved in conducting literary classes at the district level or in the villages. They may also be involved in the training of young technicians in fields where they have developed their expertise.

  It was reported that in Chongqing, a team of retired engineers had once been formed to help train 600 rural technicians working in nearby villages. Furthermore, elderly persons who are skilled in calligraphy and instrument playing are also involved in teaching these interests in various workers' and youth centres.

- Sanitary Services: In China, health and sanitary stations are set up in every district of the cities and in the villages. These stations are manned by paramedical professionals like nurses; their duties are to ensure the sanitation of their own districts or villages and to carry out simple health jobs like inoculation.

  Elderly persons are often involved in these stations as volunteers and they help in delivering medicine to the sick and supervising sanitary duties carried out in the districts and villages.

- Household Work: It is well known that the elderly in China are treasured at home not simply because of their respected position in the family but also for their contribution in household work. A survey conducted in 1985 in a village near Tianjin found that 73.1% of the elderly were the chief contributors in household work and a similar survey in Beijing found that 42% of the elderly were involved in household work to various degrees. Since more than 80% of the elderly in China are living with their married children, their contribution in household work has therefore greatly lessened the burden of the young couples and made it possible for the married women to go out to work.

CONTRIBUTION TO SOCIETY

The above represent some of the ways through which the elderly in China are involved in making their contribution towards their own families and society. As the majority of the retired workers in the cities are assured of a basic living standard by receiving old age pensions, they can serve as volunteers in various projects in which their experience and skills are still valued. As for the elderly living in the villages, their major involvement is in their households and their contribution in looking after their grandchildren and helping in household chores is very much treasured.

As China is still a developing country, jobs are available that suit the capability of the elderly and it is also the official stand that the elderly should be provided with opportunities to participate in community affairs. This has resulted in China in the development of an apparently less sophisticated welfare system in support of the elderly who are, nevertheless, compensated by the plentiful opportunities which they have in making their contributions towards the family and society (Chow, 1987).

Incentives to activity **15**

Details of a Hong Kong initiative

Alex Yui-huen Kwan

Hong Kong is one of the most densely populated places in the world. The present population of Hong Kong is estimated to be approximately 5.9 million people. Its population in mid-1990 included 748 700 people aged 60 and over (12.6%), a figure which is expected to rise to 974 500 in mid-2000 (15.1%).

Increasing numbers of older persons will result in a corresponding increase in the demand for greater number, variety and duration of services for the elderly. At the end of 1991, there were 166 social centres and 17 multi-service centres for the elderly in Hong Kong and each of these centres has provided various degrees of volunteer services by the older persons to their peers in the community. Within this review we will highlight three outstanding and well-organized elderly volunteer projects (Actualization and Reward Scheme for Senior Volunteers; Elderly Volunteer Award Scheme; and Life Enrichment Award Scheme for Elderly Volunteers) which presently exist in Hong Kong.

ACTUALIZATION AND REWARD SCHEME FOR SENIOR VOLUNTEERS

This is a territory-wide project initiated by Yan Oi Tong Woo Chung Multi-Service Centre for the Elderly in February, 1991. The objectives of the project are to promote aged volunteerism by providing financial support to assist ten elderly volunteer groups to actualize their meaningful service projects; to recognize and appreciate the contribution of the participants; and to arrange opportunities for elderly service practitioners to exchange their valuable experiences in working with elderly volunteers. At the end of one year's service, the following awards were given to respective participants (age 60+) after being screened by a panel of judges:

- outstanding elderly volunteer award
- best service project award
- the oldest volunteer award
- the highest participation award

Up to now they have mobilized more than 80 senior volunteers to provide the following activities to their peers in the community:

- fundraising for China's flood victims;
- friendly visitor for elderly staying alone;
- exchange service with elderly hostels;
- volunteer service for isolated elderly in public housing estates;
- visits to elderly homes;
- physical examination and health talk for centre's members;
- games stall on civic education fun fair;
- singing contest;
- volunteer training course;
- seminar and exhibition on health care of elderly.

ELDERLY VOLUNTEER AWARD SCHEME

The project has been organized by the Hong Kong Christian Service since April, 1990. Its objectives are acknowledging the contributions of elderly volunteers and encouraging the elderly to use their potential in servicing the community. Every year the agency will openly invite nominations for outstanding elderly volunteers (age 60+) from various social welfare agencies; then they are screened by a panel of judges according to four categories of awards (bronze, silver, gold and diamond). The criteria of awards are based on the total number of hours and the qualities of services.

Up to the end of May 1992, there were 700+ elderly volunteers enlisted in the scheme. Their services include visiting, fundraising, reception, companion, shows, shopping, physical examination, cleaning, nursing care, writing letters, hair cutting, election, instructor, household maintenance, etc.

The award scheme criteria are as follows, listing the minimum hours required and also the categories of service considered:

Diamond: 120 hours – Service attitude, co-operation,
                       problem solving, leadership
Gold: 96 hours   – Service attitude, co-operation, problem solving
Silver: 72 hours   – Service attitude, co-operation
Bronze: 48 hours   – Service attitude

LIFE ENRICHMENT AWARD SCHEME FOR ELDERLY VOLUNTEERS

This project was introduced by the Hong Kong Society for the Aged in June, 1989. The participant's age must be between 50 and 65 years old. Every year a total of 60 elderly volunteers will be recruited. The objectives of the project are:

1. to encourage pre-retirees andretireesfully to use their potential;
2. to enrich their post-retirement life;
3. to have an active and meaningful life through volunteer services to the community.

After seven sessions of basic training, participants will engage in four months' voluntary services in the community. By the end of the servicing period, they will be awarded a medal and souvenir according to the total hours of service provided (25 hours for bronze, 35 hours for silver and 45 hours for gold). So far their services include visiting, hair cutting, writing letters, assisting programmes, instructor, medical check-up, fun fair, fundraising, social gatherings, outings, interest groups, etc.

As we suggested at the beginning of this chapter, older people in Hong Kong participate in a variety of volunteer work. It is one of the mechanisms for maintaining personal ties and promoting a sense of worth. It is difficult to say what proportion of our older population is actually involved in voluntary work, for many older people have an inclination for becoming involved, without formal linkages.

The success of the above three Hong Kong programmes illustrates that older people can be quite effective in volunteer positions. But it must not be overlooked that it is undesirable to force all elderly into accepting an activity model. Furthermore, the potential for exploiting their willingness to contribute voluntarily to essential social services cannot be ignored.

Our experiences tell us that a major obstacle to the effective use of older volunteers has been an unwillingness to assign them to responsible, meaningful positions on an ongoing basis. On the other hand, many older people who are not interested in making ongoing commitments are willing to donate time and energy to one-off events or programmes that last a few weeks at most. Looking into the future, we can expect that there will be more volunteer opportunities for the senior citizen of Hong Kong to take part in and we hope that more organized efforts can be established to facilitate them even more.

Senior citizens unite 16

Pakistan Senior Citizens Association

S.M. Zaki

Less than 100 years ago, old age and retirement problems scarcely existed in the land now known as Pakistan. Families were much closer than today and it was quite normal to have three generations in one home. Grandfather was the head of the family, Grandmother helped with the upbringing of the children and the joint family system provided them with requisite shelter and maintenance, in health as well as in sickness.

Much has changed. With the fragmentation of the family unit, the problems of the elderly are becoming more acute, particularly in the big cities. Traditional family units are breaking down into 'nuclear families'. There are economic pressures, as well as personal preferences, which keep the old and ageing away from the families of their grown-up children. They are also affected by migration of the younger generation, often to distant lands, to earn a livelihood.

Demographically the percentage of over-60s in the Pakistan population is set to increase from 6.8% in 1961 to 12% in 2020. Taking youth as well as old age dependency, in 1981 Pakistan had a 95.3% dependency ratio, meaning that, on average, every working age person had one dependent person, either child or elder. And as not every working age person actually works or contributes to the national economy this is a heavy burden for a developing country to bear. Additionally, migration affects services in that, for example, a considerable proportion of doctors qualified in Pakistan have migrated to the Gulf States or the UK and are not available for local practice.

After the World Assembly on Aging, held in Vienna in 1982, the Pakistan Senior Citizens Association was formed in 1985 as a national specialized non-government organisation. The Association has as one of its central objectives the 'empowerment' of the elderly. This implies persuasion-cum-moral pressure or inducement to secure for the elderly overdue facilities and foster self-help performance.

The Pakistan Senior Citizens Association is an open membership organisation, non-partisan and independent. Representing a growing segment of the national population, it constitutes a clear single voice for stating the desires and needs of that segment. Its voice is given somewhat more authority because traditionally in Pakistan and other Islamic cultures the voice of the elder has been treated with respect. Whilst in recent years the voice of youth has tended to dominate, folk memory of the authority of the elder is still strong.

Traditionally the elder has had what might be termed the role of 'high priest' within the family. The *jirga* system of the North Western Frontier province invested the elder with considerable powers, even to the extent of imposing the death penalty in certain cases. In the *panchayat* or village council, chosen elders were the most influential group. Elders, male and female, were the chief organizers of marriages, social functions, family events and rural work programmes.

THE ASSOCIATION'S INFLUENCE

Until recently disfavour has been turned upon the direct distribution of charity to poor individuals, either by rich persons or even by the Government. It has been more acceptable for local elders to organize co-operative assistance in cases of need. Therefore the activities of the Senior Citizens Association follow in that charitable tradition, except that the persons in need are now often the elderly themselves. So it has been possible for the Association to influence national thought as a natural process, but, at the same time, good use has been made of modern publicity methods such as the press, electronic media, radio and television. The International Elderly Day has been celebrated as well as more local 'volunteer days'.

One serious consideration is the disparity between elderly males and elderly females, both in authority and living circumstances. Among older women there is a serious problem of lack of education. Excessive childbearing leads to premature ageing and lack of drive. Frequently widowhood creates a lifelong struggle where a woman with no technical skill or work history has to find ways and means of 'keeping body and soul together'. Certain taboos exist which mean that, even in better educated families, older women may be loath to participate in the activities of non-governmental organisations working for their benefit.

The fairly 'softly, softly' approach of the Senior Citizens Association has avoided alienating potential allies and has secured some notable concessions including the following:

- As a result of a civil suit in the Supreme Court the Government agreed on ethical grounds to increase retirement pensions by 32% (although not all elderly are yet eligible).
- The 1992–3 federal budget for the first time included financial provisions for senior citizens.
- A Working Group for Senior Citizens was nominated by the Government in 1987, leading to inclusion in the Social Action Plan for three years, 1992–5, of financial support for seniors' projects.
- In three (out of four) provinces, 15% of Government hospital beds have been reserved for older patients.
- 50% concessions are made to older people on official transport in two provinces.
- A 5% quota of Government programmed housing is allocated for persons in advanced age groups.
- The policy of granting loans on easy installments for self-employment programmes has been eased by the Government in respect of age limits.
- Extensions have been made to pension, as well as medical and social assistance, eligibility in all provinces.
- The introduction of Bait-Ul-Mal-Cum-Zakat, a type of state-controlled charity for the poor and needy, derived from compulsory deductions of 2.5% from the savings of Muslims – with the benefits being available also to non-Muslims.

This last innovation is very much in line with traditional Muslim tennets requiring both respect and affectionate care for all older persons as a basic right of the elder and duty of the Believer.

In the 1980s the Association noted the absence of infrastructure and of appropriately trained personnel to work on geriatric and gerontological problems. It therefore produced a research paper, which the author presented at a 1987 workshop in Islamabad. The findings of this paper, urging action to redress the lack of facilities and staff, now has official Government blessing. A priority will be to combat the so-called 'inter-generational gap', with a view to the family rather than Western type institutions being seen as the main resource in the future.

Noting the need for extensive training for Pakistan personnel in various disciplines of age care, the Senior Citizens Association took the lead in setting up seminars and workshops in various aspects and for varying levels of practitioner expertise. An epoch making event was the June 1990 Workshop for Social Workers and Senior Citizens which was planned and coordinated by the Association but fully funded by the Federal Government. International agencies have also demonstrated readiness to co-fund activities of this nature.

RECOMMENDATIONS FOR ACTION

As a result of the relatively brief but successful experience of the Pakistan Association it is possible to offer certain recommendations which might have wider application. Among these ideas are:

- A start on economic support, health, housing and social services measures at a national level for the 70 and over age group, later reducing the age limit, perhaps to 55.
- The promotion of effectively coordinated voluntary and part-time paid work by able and active elders serving more frail older people.
- Special attention to the problems of women (and also some other classes such as the terminally ill).
- More active reference to the Vienna International Plan of Action on Ageing (from the World Assembly of 1982) with the collaboration of the Federal Committee on Ageing linking to NGOs.
- Development of a National Institute of Gerontology, together with use of international consultancy.
- Replication in Pakistan of training models for carers already experimented with elsewhere.
- Opening of local age care centres to support and relieve family carers.
- Further surveys of the elderly, their circumstances, desires and needs, followed by adequate publication of information in the national language.

In view of the fact that the term 'empowerment' is being used more and more by gerontologists in some countries, a word of warning from the Pakistan experience is apposite. Leaving aside the actual dictionary definitions, it must be realised that in some Asian cultures the word can be understood as signifying 'forced' or 'arbitrary' accession to power. In certain political circles this might be construed as constituting a rather violent challenge to the current regime in power. This is obviously not intended but could be misunderstood by those who, from the seat of ultimate power, control and guide the destinies of the elderly. The Pakistan Association would find terms such as 'entitlement' or 'induce-ment' to be more sensitive and appropriate. However, this is merely a linguistic point and does not in any way detract from the Association's experience that seeking empowerment, or entitlement, or inducement, on behalf of the elderly within a nation is of the highest priority among the many options of action to meet the potential problems of a rapidly ageing population.

In Pakistan religious injunctions still have considerable influence in these times of changing attitudes, especially in intergenerational affairs. It might be good if nations revived the teachings which were the source of their cultural traditions and which inculcated respect for the elderly.

The Holy Quran has much to say in this respect, including:

Remember when we made a covenant with people of Israel and said: 'Worship no one but God and be good to your parents'.

(*Al-Baqara 83*)

Tell them: 'Come, I will read out what your Lord has made binding on you: that you make none the equal of God, and be good to your parents'.

(*Al-Anaam 151*)

So your Lord has decreed: do not worship anyone but Him and be good to your parents. If one or both of them grow old in your company, do not defy them, nor restrain them but say gentle words to them and be affectionate with them out of kindness, and say, 'O Lord, have mercy on them as they nourished me when I was small'.

(*Bani Israel 24*)

Note: On behalf of the Pakistan Senior Citizens Association, S.M. Zaki has himself prepared a substantial volume entitled *Life-Style Guide for Senior Citizens in Third World Countries.* Whilst written particularly with Pakistan and Muslim communities in mind, it is an extensive and useful work, covering many areas of concern for the elderly and suitable for direct use or adaptation in other cultures at similar stages of economic and ageing transition.

Their own counsel 17

Elderly people combine to influence their own destiny (Mexico, Australia, Argentina)

Ken Tout

A number of elderly programmes, especially in the income generating field, have drawn great benefit from the local knowledge, life experience and solid judgement of the participants, both in initial conception of ideas and in ongoing strategies. Some caring agencies have based their organization and programmes almost entirely on the elder input, as against those agencies which are initially instigated by younger groups in charge of governmental, professional or volunteer programmes.

COUNCILS OF THE ELDERLY

An early initiative in this line was a nationwide conference of elected elders in Chile in 1984 as a joint endeavour by ANIPSA, Chile and HelpAge to stimulate interest in and knowledge of elders' problems throughout the country. A continuing Mexican programme carries the title *Huehueteques* or Councils of Elders (Rangel, 1988).

The concept of the Mexican scheme is derived from the Nahuatlacas tribe of some 600 years ago which was governed at village level by Councils of Elders or Huehueteques. They were responsible for everything in the local community from law and order to the times of seed sowing and harvesting. Obviously the 1990s version only has authority over itself, but is a good example of self-governing groupings of older people.

The Mexican official federal agency responsible for elderly welfare is widely known as 'La DIF' (*sistema nacional para el Desarrollo Integral de la Familia*). It gives high priority to sponsoring local community volunteer initiatives for all age groups. One of its major tasks has been to support the growth of the Huehueteques, particularly in urban shanty areas of Mexico City which is now a vast metropolis, although the system is countrywide. DIF is always careful to indicate and encourage the full autonomy of such groups.

About 150 Councils of Elders already exist in Mexico. DIF assists in the surveys necessary to assess needs and identify appropriate geographical areas for new Councils of Elders in the very mobile new urban developments. The opinions and expertise of younger local community leaders are also invoked but the central responsibility for planning and initiating activities remains with the elders themselves. They elect their own directorate and recruit their own constituency.

Through DIF there is immediate access to all official services such as health promotion, preventive medicine, hospital and social services and rehabilitation. The programmes have a very significant cultural component as Mexicans love to relate back to earlier history and have no difficulty in identifying with the ancient native traditions, although these have been largely superseded in modern life. Drama, instrumental and choral activities are a feature of most groups.

The Councils exercise their own system of monitoring of elderly life in the community as members are able to check on the health and well-being of their peers, seeking appropriate aid for any emergency – for which information is always at hand. Whilst the majority of the Councils function in urban areas of great social need, there is an increase in their development in those rural areas where they can exercise functions more related culturally to the circumstances of the original Huehueteques.

WOMEN'S OWN

In Australia the Older Women's Network (OWN) is also an autonomous, self-generated agency springing from women's own initiatives. It is described as 'a voluntary group which takes up a wide range of issues that challenges the stereotypes of ageism and sexism . . . groups focusing on health, housing, retirement income, theatre, self-protection, guided autobiography, memory training, etc'. It is strong on mutual support, skill development and social action (Onyx et al., 1992).

OWN grew out of the Combined Pensioners Association, but this was felt by some women to be male-dominated so that a separate agency was needed to stress feminine issues. It evolved in Sydney, has spread throughout New South Wales and, more recently, has put down roots in other Australian states. Securing funding for training courses for members in 1985, the founding members set up 17 theme workshops during 1985–6. Whilst other specific grants have been gained, OWN is organized and administered by volunteers, with paid employees grant-aided for one-off projects only. However, one of the grants was for employment of an older woman to develop OWN on a national basis for the future.

The four principal objectives of OWN relate to the development of older women's skills, the strengthening of support networks, the involvement of older women in assessing their own specific needs and the dispelling of 'the invisibility of older women'. In fact it was a dramatic presentation with that same title which was put on in the open air at Canberra's Parliament House and drew considerable official and public attention to OWN. It also resulted in the formation of a permanent OWN Theatre Group.

The NSW State Government holds a 'Focus on Ageing' week and for this the OWN Theatre Group produced, as keynote events, further dramatic works entitled 'Showing Our OWN Age' and 'Women Centre Stage'. Following on the general 'Focus on Ageing' event, OWN introduced the idea of an older women's Spring Festival as a showpiece for older women's abilities and achievements. This in turn spawned a series of similar events.

On a more overtly political debate level, OWN joined with the Human Rights Equal Opportunities Commission to set up a forum on the theme 'Security and Dignity for Older Women: developing action'. It also continued to run specific workshops on subjects widely differing but of great importance to women, ranging from 'developing confidence' to 'water comfort' and 'sexuality'.

It is early yet to try to assess the impact of OWN, either on society in general or on elderly women in particular. Certainly considerable interest has been aroused and major presentations, both in publicity events and in forum recommendations, have been achieved. One of the besetting problems of OWN is the need for the substantial funding which obtains significant public action. Strangely, it has been the sad experience of OWN, which is already well known for its bold and ambitious activities for the progress and well-being of older women, that on more than one occasion applications for much needed financial support have been rejected on the grounds that OWN's own members are 'not frail enough'!

ELDERS FOR INTEGRATED DEVELOPMENT

An Argentine agency first came to the notice of international funding sources because of its excellence in developing low key income generating programmes for older persons within the community in Cordoba, a provincial capital city. It quickly proved, however, that the objectives of local agency FAIAF were much wider and more ambitious than the immediate prospect of providing a little extra income for a limited number of persons.

The Foundation for Integrated Assistance to the Elderly and the Family (FAIAF is the acronym for its Spanish title) is a non-governmental organization with interests ranging across age groups and from elders' workshops to drug addiction and 'green' issues. It is both a community activities programme and an educational awareness and lobbying campaign. It employs trained technical staff to support voluntary initiatives, with the non-technical group involved in planning its own course from the inception of an idea.

In terms of its wider work with elders its intention has been defined as that 'the elders . . . will take issue with closed institutions, those which limit older people's scope for action, or are simply assistentialist in outlook: the idea is to facilitate the participation and the integrated development of elderly people. It is nonetheless recognized that the "closed institutions" have a specific role to play in providing services for dependent elders' (Ball, 1992).

Having a remit for action across all age groups, FAIAF fully recognizes the value of intergenerational action and that elders suffer from the same attitudes and prejudices which tend to marginalize other disadvantaged groups. There is therefore some added power in FAIAF's intergenerational campaigning, but in the specific issues of ageing the elders play a particular and largely autonomous role.

Argentina's 1980 census revealed that persons over 60 years of age already constituted over 12% of the national population (a high percentage for a developing country at that time). The elder population has increased considerably, both proportionately and in gross numbers, since 1980, so that the older population can already be a significant pool of opinion, as well as skills and political support, in Argentine public life. Cordoba city itself is a concentration area for retired citizens.

The independent capability of the elder groups within FAIAF's orbit is developed in two special areas. One is that indicated already, of intervening in closed institutions and public life in general to correct erroneous perceptions of ageing and combat discriminating prejudice against the elderly. The other area of development is in self-management, a term which can include both an improved personal discipline in life and an active role in the planning, running and monitoring of community projects for the older population.

Assisted as to technicalities by FAIAF's expert staff, the elder groups, with names like *Manos Generosas* (Generous Hands), *Amor y Vida* (Love and Life) and *Jardin de la Tercera Edad* (Garden of the Third Age, appropriately located in the Magnolias district), initiate and manage almost every feasible activity in which a citizen of Cordoba might wish to become involved. These include crafts, ceramics, physical exercises and sports, drama, income earning tasks, outings and a considerable activity in art. This wide variety of interests is born out of the access that every older participant has to planning and discussion at all stages.

In 1991 a study was made of self-management in two elder groups, Manos Generosas and Armonia (Harmony). This looked at both the factors influencing the group's conception and development and also the impact of the group upon its own members.

Interim findings, as relayed by Ball, are of great interest to other similar groups in many cultures and geographical locations and the present writer would especially subscribe to the first. They include the following.

- A group which has established roots within its own community is much more likely to be effective than a project which is set up independently by an organization which has little or no base in the community.
- Using social networks as a mechanism for forming a group can be more successful than initially convening large meetings, which bring together too many people.
- The clear identification of specific objectives enables leaders to operate more effectively than leaders who have no clear concept of what they are trying to do.
- Initial technical or economic support for the implementation of a specific activity is a most important factor for the achievement of autonomy (whereas elsewhere evolving groups have sometimes regarded expert assistance as detracting from eventual autonomy).
- Loneliness and depression caused by bereavement are the most important stimuli to requirement by elders for group participation.

INITIATIVES OF OLDEST ELDERS

A smaller and more confined example of elder group involvement has been described elsewhere in this book in the section on the herbal medicine project in Vilcabamba, Ecuador (page 129). The prime lesson of the Vilcabamba committee is the ability of elders to take part in planning and conceptualization of projects at quite an advanced age.

The rural village group at Vilcabamba has a Spanish title which translates as 'the Committee for the Defence of the Old Person of Vilcabamba'. Surprisingly, that 'Defence' has been planned and carried through for some years by a committee of which at least 50% of the participants, sometimes more, have been 'Old Persons' of Vilcabamba themselves.

At the initial meeting, with the present writer in attendance, the speakers, with the exception of the local medical officer, were all of the higher age brackets. Vilcabamba people revel in their longevity and take rather a delight in somewhat exaggerating their ages, but at the same time respect is paid on a basis of a person being older. So the key speaker was a man said to be 118 years of age, although perhaps a decade younger. All spoke with considerable sense, good humour and an understanding of human affairs far beyond what would be assumed from the rural isolation of the village.

As recorded elsewhere, both the ideas and the methods for setting up a garden to produce herbal medicines came from the elders. It was a concept which was probably beyond the thought range of younger people at that time.

One instructive factor emerging from a University of Loja (Province) study in Vilcabamba underlined the danger of external experts or agencies underestimating the ability of elders from remote rural areas to discuss and plan their own destiny. Even if high in proportion of illiteracy (36%, with another 31% having only one year at school) they may have considerable artistic leanings and intellectual aptitudes. For instance, 64% owned some kind of musical instrument (percentage of the villagers over 70); 82% took part in music, dancing and other festival performances; 27% read regularly including history, medical subjects and Spanish classics; whilst over 70% made very practical proposals, often quite original, for an extension of their normal work activities if the opportunity arose (Tout, 1989).

PART SIX
Fitness and well-being

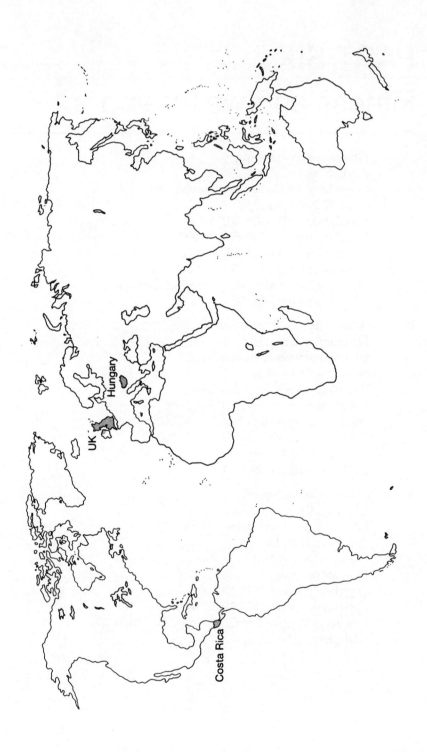

Fitness survives ageing

18

Programmes of the Costa Rican Gerontological Association (AGECO)

Zaida Esquivel

Costa Rica (meaning the Rich Coast) forms part of the Central American region and had a total population of 2 600 000 at the last census in 1984. Life expectancy at birth was 73.7 years and the group of persons over 60 constituted 6% of the population.

The ageing of human populations is a world phenomenon and Costa Rica is a part of it. We are experiencing a gradual growth in the proportion of the total population over 60 because of demographic transition in terms of the sustained reduction in the fertility rate and the increase in survival of the population. In Costa Rica this trend has a great impact on all areas of action, especially in those of employment, demand and provision of medical and social services, the consumption and production of goods and the social dynamics of the family.

It was in the years of the 1960s that the rapid decline in fertility rates commenced, bringing on the ageing of the population. As to the future, according to the forecasts, the process of ageing will be intensified until, by the year 2025, Costa Rica will have reached the same levels of greying as Europe and North America, with as much as 24% of the population aged 70 and more.

In studying the distribution of older persons by sex, it is notable the extent by which the female group exceeds the male; for instance, in the over-80 band there are currently some 10 753 females compared to only 7 721 males. In brief, Costa Rica expects the over-60s population to double within 19 years.

In respect of demand for services it is also of note that although the over-60s group as yet represents only 6.4% of the population, the group accounts for 11.8% of hospital admissions and 13% of medical consultations. Different studies carried out in the country indicate that the proportion of elders who live alone does not exceed 10%. Another 3% reside in institutions. So the majority continue to be integrated into families although now a certain amount of family rejection is becoming evident.

With respect to income, we find that in the case of men the principal source is pensions which benefit some 45% of males. Wages received for continuing work are received by 35%. In the case of women aged from 60 to 64 the main source is support from children, although for women over 65 pensions come to occupy the first place. But if we remember that the pensions are low amounts we can see that there does exist a major problem of subsistence.

In addition to the above details it is important to mention the following points.

- We know that the Costa Rican population is increasing at a very fast rate.
- Of the aged population, a high percentage still live with the family but there exist significant signs of change in the family structure and, above all, in the attitude of the family towards its elders, with daily reports of a certain level of abuse to elders.
- There has been noted a strong proliferation of centres for elders, both public and private profit centres, which leads us to believe that there is a great demand for this type of service.

WHAT IS AGECO?

The *Asociacion Gerontologica Costarricense* (AGECO) is a non-governmental organisation and non-profit making. It was founded in 1980 with the object of improving the quality of life of the elderly. The aims of AGECO, as laid down in its statues, are:

1. to study the problem of the Third Age and the solutions which may be appropriate so that this social group may enjoy a dignified old age in keeping with its human rights, both in personal aspects and with the family and society;
2. to promote, study and take part in activities directed to obtaining policy definitions and the promulgation of legal measures which may be required for the Third Age and to watch for their fulfilment;
3. to create an awareness in the community and in individuals belonging to this social group as to their human and intellectual value during the Third Age.

AGECO STRATEGIES AND POLICIES

These are in keeping with the recommendations of the World Assembly on Ageing which recognizes that the quality of life is no less important than longevity and that consequently older persons ought, as far as possible, to enjoy a full, healthy, secure and satisfying life and should be recognized as an integral part of society. So the programmes take the line of education, promotion, training and development for persons of the Third Age, as well as for their family, community and society in general.

AGECO takes great pains so that older people may assume their positive role in society and attain a level of high value and respect. It combats the paternalistic attitude that tends to make elders dependent and favours ways in which they can become social activists responsible for their own destiny. In its daily dealings AGECO orientates its activities in the four areas of training and technical support; prevention and education; promotion and organization; and services.

The area of training and technical assessment counts with an inter-disciplinary technical group which provides these means of support to old people's homes and day centres. There are support groups organized in the community and the various institutions to provide theoretical and practical skills which will improve the quality of life of the old person both in institutions and in the community.

The area of prevention and education commences with a campaign of information through the mass media. It has as its aim the raising of awareness and knowledge of the public, as well as the humanizing of the society in which we live. It seeks to construct positive images of ageing and the aged and to modify the stereotypes and activities leading to marginalization.

Knowing the important role which the media can play, AGECO has a constant campaign with the press, television and radio seeking to teach people how to age and avoid risks; to maintain respect for the elderly; and to teach those who are already elderly how to organize themselves and fight for the right to have an active and full life.

Then there is the Youth Campaign directed at pupils in primary schools with the objective of strengthening intergenerational relation-ships by teaching children the realities of ageing. This programme has a coverage of about 55 000 children for whom special educational stories are published. A particular success in this respect was when a strip cartoon, teaching about relationships with grandparents and prepared for the campaign, was seen by a national newspaper and found to be fascinating and professionally well-designed. The strip now appears weekly in the national press.

Also in this sector are included courses for the elders and for family carers. For the elders the courses deal with developing positive attitudes, increasing self-esteem and generating new ways of using free time. There are four such courses each year. For family carers the courses specialize in self-care, independent living, autonomy of choice and direct care.

The range of activities is supported by AGECO's own publications, which have various themes such as health or psychosocial matters, for example, *Practical Advice for the Third Age, Disciplined Exercise, Adaptations for Centres Attending to the Elder* as well as monthly bulletins, press releases and so on.

The area of promotion and organization is concerned very much with health promoting, fitness preserving activities for the elderly themselves.

The Ecology Project, taking advantage of current ecological interest, was mounted in the search to find new opportunities in which the elderly might assume a more active role in society. This project, which is a pilot project as yet, is being developed in collaboration with the International Union for the Conservation of Nature, with a sharing of human and economic resources. This first elders' nature conservation group will have a role in educating and practically guarding the riches of nature with the elders as 'watchdogs'.

Recreational activities are an area in which AGECO has been a pioneer. There is a multiplicity of diverse activities through which the elders assume a more positive attitude, develop greater interest in current events and improve their physical and mental condition. Important among these is *Hydroquinesia* in which the participants do physical exercises in water. There are also many outings to places of cultural and tourist interest.

Since 1987 AGECO has organized an annual road race of the Third Age with people over 60 taking part, which attracts much public interest as well as stimulating the elders to regular training. In offering swimming classes and facilities to urban elders who have migrated from rural areas, AGECO makes this sport available to people who have never before had the time or opportunity for swimming as health-giving leisure.

On the National Day of the Elder there takes place a 'Recreational and Cultural Festival' between competing centres of the Third Age. In this gathering all manner of games, competitions and cultural presentations take place, with the elders in charge of events, competing with all seriousness but also with great enjoyment.

The Programme of Volunteers, which was launched in 1991, is directed at the recruitment of a group of persons, themselves of the Third Age, who have an interest in dedicating their free time to the service of other people and groups who are more needy. There was no hesitation in volunteering and already a group of 60 persons is actively developing support programmes in institutions for the needy elderly, institutions for children, institutions of support for adolescent single mothers, museums and rehabilitation centres. This group of elderly volunteers has received an ample training in accordance with the area of work undertaken and there also exists a plan of continuing education as well as review and assessment of the group's work.

Alternative Third Age Clubs are being developed to seek the most appropriate ways of catering for the needs of older people in the community, again concentrating on the reintegration of the elders and their opportunities for sufficient socializing. The regular contact and social interchange, if nothing else, already serve to reduce the marginalization and isolation of people of the Third Age. The clubs are conceived of not as services to the elders but as services with and of the elders, with a self-generating productivity in all fields, cultural, social and economic. The clubs have clear objectives:

- to offer a new alternative in social interchange and bring maximum benefit from use of spare time;
- to reduce the feeling of loneliness and isolation;
- to promote physical and psychological well-being of the members and then further develop their undiscovered physical and mental potential.

On the mental aspect it has been possible to introduce older people from apparently poor educational and cultural origins into full involvement in specialist clubs on music, reading of classics, theatre, dance and so on. In the physical realm there are also clubs which concentrate entirely on gymnastics, swimming, yoga and various sports.

In addition to these specialist groups, to which any older person can belong, there are the community clubs, strategically located for easy access, but each of which offers an entire range of less specialist activities, as well as introduction to the specialist groups. Useful crafts are encouraged especially where there is an urgent need for older persons to supplement their income.

The role of AGECO with the Third Age Clubs is that of promoter and facilitator rather than owner. AGECO does not seek to set up a monopoly of national clubs. It works through the commitment of local community leaders, but often the first commitment of AGECO is to create awareness in local leaders in districts where perhaps the evidence of a greying population, and of dire need within that group, is not yet at what might be termed 'crisis level'. So members of AGECO staff will visit a 'new' community to motivate interested local persons and to assess what the strength of potential support is likely to be.

AGECO has a useful and successful format of assessment and promotion in a new district, with a special focus on aspects such as the objectives, programmes and activities of AGECO itself; the importance, benefits and specific functioning of the clubs; systems of community organisation; leadership as related to work with elders; group dynamics.

Having acted in the roles of promoter, motivator, facilitator and assessor to new clubs AGECO then, once a club is set up, offers its expert visiting service to help monitor and evaluate the working of the club, always with the aim of making the participants in the new venture autonomous and capable of establishing and maintaining their own systems as locally and culturally appropriate.

Invariably this approach results in clubs desiring a continuing link into AGECO and a monthly meeting of club coordinators takes place in the AGECO offices. Through this meeting many of the special and united events, social, recreational and cultural, can be planned and coordinated throughout the year.

There are now regular media programmes for the elderly on which information and announcements can be made known. Among these are, for instance, National Radio's 'Grandparents' Box' on Thursday mornings, *La Nacion* newspaper's Golden Age column every Monday and Radio Reloj's 'Social Service' programme daily. All these will take either national or local announcements of events great or small.

The internal government of each club is democratic. Members discuss their own specific targets and plans and also elect a Coordinator on an annual basis. They also carry out their own internal monitoring and evaluation with regard to achievement of their own stated objectives.

There is within the extensive national network of clubs so far established its own multiplication factor. Already the network is an effective national information exchange which reaches out through the media to districts and cultural groups which have so far not developed a similar programme. In a more casual way, by word of mouth, older people in unserviced areas develop their own ambition to set up a club and apply to AGECO for the initial guiding hand.

Public service is another AGECO activity which is of major use to members of the clubs, but is also available to family carers of the general public. There is a 'Bank of Aid Equipment'. This is a store of useful aids such as wheelchairs, air cushions, bath seats, orthopaedic aids and so on. Expensive to purchase for a short period, these aids can be lent or hired to elders or carers as needed.

Another public service is the 'Centre of Documentation', an AGECO reference library on geriatrics and gerontology. This contains some 700 publications and also has subscriptions to seven prominent specialist bulletins. It is in constant use, demand for its services is growing and a computerized system is being developed and will shortly be in use. Commercial firms also call in AGECO to run preretirement courses for workers who have no concept of what retirement is.

Perhaps it should be pointed out that AGECO was not, at its foundation, an association of qualified geriatricians. It arose from the initiatives of a group of concerned citizens from many differing walks of life, with a civil engineer as its president. There was always available a cadre of geriatric and gerontological experts for advice to the voluntary and non-specialist governing body, although that body did itself include members with considerable expertise in areas such as business organization, publicity, economics and education.

The results so far can be defined as most encouraging. The work done in various areas is bearing visible fruit, AGECO has the active backing and support of the mass of elders and communities, who have themselves evolved into effective multipliers and publicists of the programmes.

Perhaps the most serious problems were encountered at the very start of the initiative and were generated within AGECO itself, in the form of serious trepidation about whether self-motivation and activity of older people would work. Old stereotypes were hard to lay to rest. We needed to convince ourselves that the Third Age **can** and that the Third Age **generates**.

Success is seen in that, at first contact, needy older people no longer ask us 'What are you going to give us?', 'What are you giving away?' Rather the response now is 'What can we do?', or 'How can we help?' Another concrete area of success has been the vast interest shown by the media where, almost without exception, all sections are actively seeking out new ways of promoting the concept of an active, productive and healthy old age. Expensive media spaces are offered free of cost and often at key moments on television.

Within AGECO itself the original governing group from all walks of life is now supported by a self-evolved small team of professional, highly skilled workers who perform with great vision and often with self-denial in their delight to see the continuing rapid growth in numbers of elderly people who join up with what is essentially a self-generating movement of the Third Age.

A foundation for good health

19

Self health care and older people

Miriam Bernard (UK)

As the contributions to this book show, effective community development work with older people can be found in many countries of the world. Even where there are substantial levels of publicly provided services this is often complemented, as in the UK, by an active and, at times, innovative independent sector. In the UK, voluntary organizations have been at the forefront of developments for older people. The variety of schemes and projects which now exist can be seen as, on the one hand, a direct response to the changing demographic picture and, on the other, as a counter to the problem orientated notion we have of old age.

Where our older people are stereotyped as roleless and redundant, one counter is through the development of programmes which have as their goal the empowerment of older people. This chapter describes the work of one British voluntary organization, the Beth Johnson Foundation.

THE DEVELOPMENT OF THE FOUNDATION

In 1972, following the death of Beth Johnson, a charitable trust was set up bearing her name. Her will provided for the whole of her estate to be used for charitable purposes and it was decided to set up the Foundation as a memorial to her. Unusually, rather than just providing sums of money to help the poor and needy, the policy of the Foundation has been to sponsor and encourage innovative work aimed at improving the quality of life for all older people. The Foundation is based in Stoke-on-Trent in north Staffordshire.

Under the guidance of a fulltime Director and a Principal Officer (Development), the Foundation initiates and supports a range of projects.

From its earliest days, it has attempted to establish activities which then become self-supporting when the Foundation withdraws its initial financial outlay. This has allowed the core staff to continue to move on and develop new projects in response to the needs expressed by the older people with whom they are in contact.

During the 1970s, the Foundation sponsored the development of what might now be regarded, in some circles, as 'conventional' schemes for older people. Set in a historical context, though, some of these developments were in fact highly innovative. For example, the Foundation sponsored the creation of an over-60s day centre; a mobile day centre serving elderly people living in remote rural areas; and neighbourhood support schemes for elderly mentally infirm people and their relatives. In addition, in 1976, the Beth Johnson Housing Association was formed. This voluntary organization is now constitutionally separate from the Foundation but retains strong links. The Beth Johnson Housing Group, as it has become, is responsible for managing and developing sheltered housing for elderly people and for a range of social housing aimed at meeting the needs of other client groups.

Throughout the 1980s, the emphasis of the Foundation's work shifted much more towards the encouragement of projects based on peer and self-help. In 1982, for example, the Beth Johnson Leisure Association was established. This still flourishing organization, with some 600 members in 1991, provides a regular programme of sports and social activities throughout north Staffordshire. It is managed by the members and its range of activities are led, for the most part, by older people themselves. This is also the basis on which the Beth Johnson Senior Centre runs. Originally located in a converted city centre church, it is now housed in club premises belonging to the Catholic Church and offers a wide programme of both sedentary and more energetic activities. Users can also obtain refreshments and a hot midday meal.

Finally, in 1984 and 1985, in partnership with the Centre for Health and Retirement Education in London, the Foundation also began to explore ways of enhancing the skills of older people in order to enable them to engage in individual counselling and support work with their peers (Bernard and Ivers, 1986; Ivers and Meade, 1991). This Peer Health Counselling Project, as it was known, was the forerunner of the Self Health Care in Old Age programme.

Alongside these practical initiatives, the Foundation has long been involved in extending knowledge about ageing and old age through its educational and research work. It has sponsored courses and seminars aimed at those working with older people in a variety of professions, as well as promoting educational activities for older people themselves. The 29 books and nine research reports published since 1976 are eloquent testimony to the Foundation's activity in these fields.

We now turn to consider one particular project which encapsulates the approach and philosophy of the Foundation: the Self Health Care in Old Age Programme.

HEALTH AND WELL-BEING IN OLD AGE

Over the last decade, there has been a growing interest in the UK in health issues and older people. Various national campaigns have come and gone, emphasizing the benefits of sport and exercise and advocating the adoption of 'healthy lifestyles', through such means as giving up smoking and changing one's diet. However, much of this kind of health education and promotion work is aimed at individuals. This can be problematic because, although on the face of it, it might appear to give individuals control over their own health, it can very easily lead to victim blaming. Such campaigns have also been criticized for diverting attention away from the structural causes of ill health and for failing to address the very practical issues which arise in translating health promotion into concrete action. However, despite these criticisms, it is noticeable that activity around this issue has undoubtedly increased and that older people have been a key group behind these developments (Bernard and Phillipson, 1991).

Self health care practices are crucial to the maintenance of health and well-being in later as well as in earlier life. It was in recognition of this fact that the Foundation, in collaboration with the (then) Health Education Council and the Department of Adult and Continuing Education at Keele University, mounted two national seminars in the mid-1980s to explore health issues in old age (Glendenning, 1985, 1986). At this time too, the Foundation, with co-funding from the European Community's Second Poverty Programme, was able to initiate its own Self Health Care in Old Age Programme.

This project did not emerge out of the blue. Rather, it evolved from the years of work with older people described above; work which had long been concerned with exploring how best people could be supported and encouraged in the pursuit of various activities designed to maintain, and indeed improve, the quality of their lives in old age.

Whilst the programme has obviously evolved and changed during the six years it has been in existence, its overall aims and objectives remain firmly rooted in the notions of empowerment, peer and self-help. Self-empowered health behaviour is a cumulative process and has to be built around a number of key factors (Hopson and Scally, 1981). These include:

- **awareness** – of one's own worth and uniqueness; of the needs and feelings of others; and of the ways in which our systems and structures can depower, or empower, individuals;

- **goals** – that one works out for oneself and that one is committed to;
- **values** – that one is clear about and that are consistent with one's goals and plan of action;
- **information** – of all kinds;
- **health and lifeskills** – that one acquires and develops and that in turn feed back into the other factors.

The staff of the Foundation also consider two additional factors to be of importance for self-empowered health behaviour amongst older people. In recognition of the fact that it can often be very difficult to change or modify the habits of a lifetime and that many older people may lack the confidence to initiate changes, it is necessary to ensure that there is adequate:

- **access** – including physical access to facilities or services; to written information; to a range of advice; and to opportunities which allow them to confront and explore their feelings about health in old age;
- **support** – both peer and professional, to translate the goals one has identified into action; and to give encouragement or support on a one-to-one basis or in a group setting.

THE SELF HEALTH CARE IN OLD AGE PROGRAMME

These seven factors are to be found in operation in the Self Health Care in Old Age Programme, whose overall aim is to provide an accessible, attractive and popular means of furthering health education and promotion amongst older people. In addition, its three specific objectives are:

1. to raise older people's awareness of the need for health care maintenance;
2. to encourage the involvement of more older people in health care programmes;
3. to assist older people to identify the skills and strategies they require to meet their health needs.

Four practical and interrelated means have been developed in order to achieve these aims and objectives. These are:

1. a Peer Health Counselling Scheme;
2. a telephone link service (CareLine);
3. a variety of health related courses/activities;
4. a Senior Health Shop.

We now consider each in turn.

PEER HEALTH COUNSELLING

The origin of this project was noted above and, in 1985, the Foundation initiated an experimental training programme which offered a number of older people the opportunity to enhance their skills in the areas of group leadership and counselling. At its simplest, Peer Health Counsellors are older volunteers who help and support other older people in matters relating to the maintenance of health and well-being.

Over the past seven years, a whole range of work has been undertaken, many new volunteers trained and an ongoing programme of regular Counsellor support and training developed. Peer Health Counsellors have been and continue to be involved in a variety of activities including:

- individual counselling and support to help people (re)establish their confidence; and to (re)introduce them to healthy lifestyle practices such as diet, exercise and stress management strategies;
- group work in institutional settings through leading gentle exercise, relaxation and health discussion groups;
- information giving at health fairs, exhibitions and conferences;
- advocacy work with frail older people in hospital settings and in residential and nursing homes;
- reminiscence therapy, in partnership with local museum and library services, for older people in a variety of settings.

They also run the telephone link service detailed below.

CARELINE

Some of the Peer Health Counsellors involve themselves in the operation of CareLine, a project which maintains contact with frail and house-bound older people by means of a telephone-out service. Counsellors have been trained in telephone counselling techniques and, each afternoon, they contact lists of older people who are deemed to be isolated and/or 'at risk'. The aims are to check on the health and well-being of clients; to monitor whether or not they have eaten, slept, taken pre-scribed drugs, etc. and to give them some contact with the outside world.

Clients are referred by professionals such as social workers, health visitors, community nurses and doctors, or by people such as informal carers, friends and neighbours. Two CareLines, each able to take up to 40 clients at a time, are now in operation, one based in the Senior Health Shop and the other in a Social Services office. The locations are important, because they mean that back-up is available from a professional worker should it be required. In addition, each client has a named key person (e.g. a relative, social worker) who can be contacted in the event that the elderly client fails to answer the telephone. Community police are also involved and will, as a final safety net, go and investigate should the Peer Health Counsellors not be able to reach either the client or the key person.

HEALTH COURSES AND ACTIVITIES

These courses and activities are mostly run under the auspices of the Leisure Association and the Senior Centre (see above). People can be referred to a whole range of health enhancing activities including yoga, swimming, rambling, badminton, keep fit, bowling, dancing, art, craft, musical and educational activities. Energetic social committees organise seasonal events as well as outings to places of interest and to the theatre and, on occasion, arrange holidays.

Specific health related courses have also been initiated as a direct result of the project. Nutrition classes and stress management classes have featured, as has the continuing and highly successful 'Look After Yourself' programme. This programme combines physical exercise with relaxation and discussions of various health topics. The exercise element is tailored to individual needs and participants are taught to monitor their own condition and to exercise within their personal capabilities.

SENIOR HEALTH SHOP

This has been the focus for the whole programme since its opening in 1986. It is literally the 'shop window' on the project and on the variety of other activities which are linked to it. Customers can find a comprehensive stock of health literature displayed around the walls that they can browse through while having refreshments from the healthy eating cafeteria. The shop is bright and attractive, is easily accessible (close to the city centre shopping precinct and the bus station) and is open to anyone over the age of 50.

Shop staff, volunteers and Peer Health Counsellors are present to discuss health issues with visitors and to advise on suitable activities, diet and exercise programmes for older people. Blood pressure checking and weight monitoring services are also available and, on occasion, professional health workers will spend time in the Shop talking to and answering questions from customers. Accessibility, appropriate support and extensive information are the key factors in the success of the Shop's operation. In 1991, the Shop attracted in excess of 10 000 visitors and it is encouraging to note that the Self Health Care Programme (in whole and in part) continues to be replicated in other areas of the country.

These four interrelated projects are directed at encouraging more positive attitudes towards health in old age. For older individuals, the programme offers help and support in the development of a healthy lifestyle; for professionals it is both a resource and, hopefully, a challenge to some of the preconceived and stereotypical notions that prevail about older people; and for policy makers it suggests alternative ways of tackling the impoverishment and disadvantage that afflicts the lives of many people in later life. Ultimately, in the prevailing climate of consumer choice and empowerment, a programme of this nature is about enabling older people to challenge the existing ways in which services are constructed and delivered. It also helps give them the confidence and skills to ask for the types of health and social care they themselves most need and want, rather than just being fitted in to what is currently on offer.

INITIATIVES FOR THE 1990s

All the projects mentioned above continue to flourish as we move further into the last decade of this century. Some, such as the Leisure Association, have become self-sustaining; others, like the Senior Centre, are still underpinned by the resources of the Foundation itself; while yet others, such as the Senior Health Shop, have attracted funding from alternative sources. In the latter case, the local Health Authority and the County Social Services Department have agreed to provide funds from Joint Finance to ensure its continuation up until 1999.

Since 1990, the role of Peer Health Counsellors has been extended and developed into an advocacy project for older people. Funded initially by the Department of Health's 'Opportunities for Volunteering' scheme, the project seeks to recruit, train, supervise and support volunteer citizen advocates. Advocates come from a wide variety of backgrounds and act as individual representatives for older people who need assistance. They work in partnership, providing emotional support through friendship and enabling the elderly person to obtain the resources and services they need to improve their quality of life. To date, most partnerships have originated in hospital settings although the work is now widening to other institutions such as nursing and residential homes and is even, on occasion, used by elderly people living in their own homes. An Advocacy Training and Support Officer coordinates the work and supports the volunteers.

Another strand of the Foundation's current activity relates to reminiscence therapy. Under the supervision of a Support Worker, trained volunteers work together in groups with older people in a variety of institutional settings such as residential homes, sheltered housing complexes and day centres. Reminiscence is important for mental health and well-being in later life and is of value to older people and those who work with them for a variety of reasons. First, it can enhance the elderly person's sense of identity and self-worth by highlighting the assets and positive experiences they bring to old age. Second, in group settings it can encourage and stimulate social exchange. Third, it can help staff by opening up new ways of communicating and, by emphasizing people's achievements and joys, it can help counter some of the negative perceptions they might hold. Finally, it moves the older person centre-stage, reversing the usual relationship and enabling older people to be active contributors of their past experience and knowledge, as opposed to the passive recipients of care.

From 1993, yet another project is planned. With matched funding from charity projects and the Foundation, a three-year programme entitled SCIPS: Senior Citizens Involved in Public Services, is to be initiated. This project aims to recruit, train and support a core group of volunteers who will be attempting to motivate older people to become more involved in the direct planning of services in their local communities. External monitoring and evaluation of the project is also proposed.

CONCLUSION

Over the 20 years of its existence, the Foundation has developed a set of underlying principles and values which it believes are key to successful community development work with older people. First, rather than viewing older people as passive recipients of care, there is an acknowledgement that given appropriate encouragement, training and support, they have a wealth of skills and experience which can be enhanced and built upon just as well in later as in earlier life.

Second, while there are some obvious dangers in overstating the idea of self-help, in the sense that it might be seen as a way for statutory services to abrogate responsibility for older people, it is vital to the process of self-empowerment. This in turn is linked with ideas around peer help as a way of facilitating this process. In this way, older people gain the confidence to challenge the prevalent and negative stereotyping to which they are subjected.

Third, peer and self-help initiatives are a complement to, rather than a replacement for, professional care. The Foundation recognizes this and, as a consequence, has worked very closely with the local Health Authority, the Social Services Department and the Local Authority in the developments it has set up in recent years.

Finally, it is important that such work is properly monitored and evaluated, for the benefit of the organization itself, for funders and for the people who both use and are directly affected by its developments. The Foundation has a strong commitment to research, believing that it is a worthwhile undertaking and one which enhances the evolution of a group or project. It is in these ways that the Foundation continues to try and help improve the quality of life for people in old age.

ACKNOWLEDGEMENTS

I wish to thank my former colleagues at the Beth Johnson Foundation, Stoke-on-Trent, England; and all the older people and volunteers who, over the years, have contributed so much to the projects and groups mentioned here.

Advised to live longer **20**

Advisory Service of the Gerontology Centre, Semmelweis (University of Medicine, Budapest)

István A. Gergely

The Gerontology Centre of the Semmelweis University of Medicine, Budapest, was founded in 1965. In the beginning it functioned as a Research Department of Gerontology and in 1978 became the Gerontology Centre. Practically since its foundation it has been directed by Professor Edit Beregi MD, DMSc, who has been elected as president of the International Association of Gerontology from 1993. The name of the Institute has been brought into repute principally by immunohistological, humoral immunological, intestinal absorption and bone metabolism experiments, longitudinal/follow-up examinations on healthy old people, epidemiological and centenarian studies. These have particularly been aimed at the better understanding of external and internal factors influencing longevity and of risk factors having a part in the development of diseases of old age.

PROGRAMME OF EXAMINATIONS

Beside the various experimental laboratories – histochemistry, immunology, biology, biochemistry, electrophysiology – and the neuropsychiatric research laboratory, the Clinical Department plays an important and decisive role in the Gerontology Centre. At the Clinical Department voluntary health screening type non-invasive examinations are being carried out in healthy older people over the retirement age, which in Hungary is 55 for women and 60 for men.

On completion of the examinations the subjects are given a report and detailed recommendations regarding the possibly necessary treatments, complementary investigations and the suggested regime of living. It is worth mentioning that only about 30% of people who consider themselves healthy prove to be really healthy, i.e. have no diseases that require treatment. With a view to studying the process of physiological ageing, the examinations are repeated on average at two or three year intervals. Up to 30th June 1992, 8238 clinical check-ups of nine days each had been carried out using the 15 beds of the Clinical Department and 1419 persons have been examined 2–13 times.

The programme of the examination is predetermined and uniform. It includes, beside the general and internal medicine investigation, the examinations of the neuropsychiatrist, ophthalmologist, oto-rhino-laryngologist, urologist and gynaecologist, laboratory, X-ray, ECG and pulmonary function tests, which are from time to time supplemented by other investigations. On the basis of the results of the check-ups, subjects are selected who are regarded as controls, e.g. for centenarian studies, or asked to participate in certain scientific projects, e.g. in immunogenetics and bone mineral content measurements, undertaken by the Gerontology Centre and other institutes.

The researchers of the Gerontology Centre regularly report on their experiences and results at domestic and international meetings and in scientific periodicals. They often give health educational and popular science lectures in clubs and institutions of the elderly and on TV and radio programmes, especially in the fields of the biology and psychology of the ageing process, diseases frequent in old age, social and health care problems of the elderly and ways of preserving health during ageing.

ELDERS HEALTH ADVISORY SERVICE

The Advisory Service has been functioning in the Gerontology Centre since 1971. For organising and operating it, Eva Lengyel MD, specialist in internal medicine, deserves almost exclusive credit. Her excellent personality, empathy, commitment to the interests of the aged, comprehensive knowledge in all areas of gerontology and indefatigable working capacity have been the basis of the successful work of the Advisory Service.

The Advisory Service functions as follows. At regular intervals, twice a month, for two or two and a half hours elderly people gather in the auditorium of the Gerontology Centre. They publicly raise questions which are, as at a briefing, promptly answered by Dr Lengyel or, in her exceptional absence, myself.

The general way and purpose of responding is that the reply be interesting and illuminating, not only for the person who has asked the question but also for the other 30 to 40 people who are present. During such an advisory meeting about 15 to 20 questions are usually answered. The questions cover all areas of healthy ways of living, diseases of old age and psychological and social problems of the elderly.

Evidently in such circumstances there is no opportunity to talk over special personal problems and complaints; these lie outside the scope of the advisory service. However, if this kind of question is put, information is given on the general implications of the issue, e.g. if somebody asks for medical advice on how to treat his or her constipation, we speak in general terms about the possible causes of constipation in old age, about the importance of a fibre-rich diet and the regime stimulating intestinal mobility, or about the various kinds and effects of laxatives and recommend to the enquirer where to go for further help and information. Some people are advised to contact our Clinical Department. There are several questions that emerge time and time again; the problems of the day concerning the elderly and the health and social care system almost regularly come into question. It happens quite frequently that someone has heard or read of something somewhere and wishes to learn the opinion of the meeting leader about it.

Raising, answering and discussing the questions occurs in an entirely informal, club-like manner. It is not uncommon that following a reply, a mostly regular participant of the meeting, other than the one who asked the question, tells the group his or her own experience or opinion. This is properly evaluated by the specialist afterwards.

THE RECURRENT WORRIES

To give a taste of the recurrent topics, the most frequent questions are the following:

- What are the causes of atherosclerosis?
- What is the significance of the high cholesterol level?
- What is the normal cholesterol level?
- What does HDL cholesterol mean?
- Does calcium intake result in atherosclerosis or arthrosis?
- What is osteoporosis?
- Why are diuretics given in high blood pressure?
- Is potassium always necessary with diuretics?
- Is coffee dangerous for hypertensive patients?
- What is Alzheimer's disease?
- What can be done against forgetfulness, insomnia, obesity, varicosity, headache, articular pain, back pain, constipation, dryness of the skin, cold feet, numbness, greying, becoming bald, shakiness, weakness, losing weight, anaemia, iron deficiency, diabetes?

- Does high sugar intake result in diabetes?
- How to stop smoking?
- Is acupuncture really effective?
- How effective are various paramedical therapeutic regimes?
- Why is salt dangerous?
- How much water is needed for a person a day?

Attention may then turn to AIDS, transfusions, minerals, vitamins, healthy diet, activity, inactivity, working capacity of the old, sport for the elderly, third age university, rights of the seniors, health insurance, pension systems, air pollution, security, chronic wards, nursing homes, sheltered housing, rehabilitation, tourism, television programmes, behaviour of the younger generations, etc.

Sometimes very special questions are asked:

- How does the pacemaker work?
- How are renal stones extracted without surgery?
- What is colonoscopy?
- What is ERCP (endoscopic retrograde choledochopancreatography)?
- Does aluminium consumption result in dementia?
- Can Parkinson's disease be treated surgically?
- What is the indication of heart transplantation?
- What does a given laboratory or other finding mean?
- What is the medicine which has been prescribed to a family member abroad?

When any new remedy or cosmetic preparation arrives on the market and is widely advertised in the media, e.g. anticholesterol pills, hair restorers, slimming capsules, multivitamin products, antiwrinkle cream, a query comes from the floor without delay. The more recent and fashionable paramedical products, of which one or two new ones appear fortnightly now in Hungary, come into question almost immediately. If there is any change, for instance, in the rules of prescribing certain drugs in the frame of the health insurance system or in the organization of community care or in the structure of the pension system, the first questions concerning the matter come soon. In such cases often no authentic answer is expected, but rather understanding and sympathy.

If sometimes an unusual question occurs that cannot entirely be responded to immediately, it will be answered next time. It may happen that a specialist co-worker of the Gerontology Centre is invited to present a 10 to 15 minutes lecture on an up-to-date topic, e.g. the immunization project against tetanus of the elderly.

Regardless of whether it has been asked for or not, Dr Lengyel regularly summarizes the most recent results of age research, gives information about the changes and the problems in the Hungarian social and health care systems and reports on the most important experiences and interesting results of domestic and international meetings in gerontology.

It is evident that definite recommendations concerning medicines cannot be given without medical examination, and mentioning names of the various products, especially comparing them to each other, should be avoided. The person raising the question often would like to know whether his or her medication is right or not. Those kinds of questions are answered only in a general way, so that the patient's trust in his doctor and the treatment may not to be affected. If necessary, the patient will be directed to the appropriate institute (it may be our own Clinical Department) so as to be properly examined or treated.

SPREADING THE WORD

The participants primarily are informed about the existence, place and time of the Advisory Service through reports and interviews given to the press and the media and from lectures held in clubs and institutions by the researchers of the Gerontology Centre. Many elderly people obtain knowledge of it from friends, neighbours or relatives.

Patients who have been investigated in the Clinical Department are also enthusiastic propagandists of the Advisory Service and, vice versa, those who frequently attend the Advisory Service often join in the longitudinal programme of the Clinical Department. There are many who come more than once and some who regularly attend the meetings, regardless of whether they have questions or not. All are eager to know what is news in gerontology and in popular science.

Some of them arrive an hour before the programme starts and stay there long after it, to meet old friends or get acquainted with new ones from the Clinical Department or the Advisory Service itself. Sometimes close friendship develops from these acquaintances; if someone becomes bedridden, others go to see that person and, if necessary, they help one another.

As volunteer organizers, they make propaganda for the Clinical Department, ensuring new subjects to select from for the longitudinal studies. There are a few men and women (the usual male/female ratio of participants is about one to three or one to four) who have attended the Advisory Service more or less regularly for two decades. In 1992 a very faithful visitor, a fine old lady, celebrated her hundredth birthday in the auditorium with the participants and the faculty and staff of the Gerontology Centre.

According to our experiences, the effect of the Advisory Service is greater than one would expect from simply giving good advice to the old people who are present. Those who frequently or regularly attend the meetings in most instances are the ones who also go to third age universities, seniors' clubs, tourists' clubs, bridge saloons, religious communities, etc. and they devotedly make publicity not only for the Gerontology Centre but also for the healthy way of living in old age, prevention of diseases of the old and last, but not least, tolerance towards others and especially the younger generations.

Not infrequently, the above mentioned organizations or communities invite a speaker from the Gerontology Centre to give a lecture on the current problems of old age.

It is due to all this that perhaps every fourth or fifth person of the 400 000 people over 60 in Budapest may greet Dr Eva Lengyel and the staff of the Gerontology Centre of the Semmelweis University of Medicine as old acquaintances when meeting them in the street, at a club or at media events.

PART SEVEN
Income generation

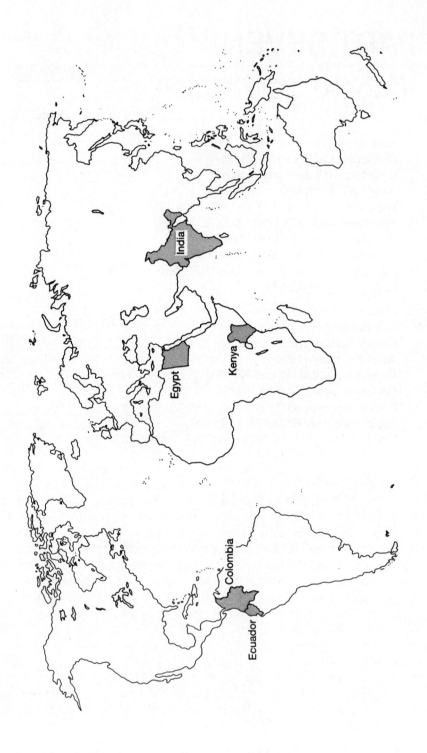

Activity, its own medicine

21

A 'Valley of the Aged' Project, Vilcabamba, Ecuador

Guillermo del Pozo V

Vilcabamba, variously known as 'The Valley of the Aged' or 'The Island of Immunity', came to world notice through a Reader's Digest article by Dr Eugene H. Payne in 1959. It was again featured in the reports by Dr Alexander Leaf on his research into the links between cholesterol and heart disease there in 1971. It was calculated at the time that, whilst in Ecuador as a whole only 4.6% of the population were over 60 years of age, in Vilcabamba the proportion was 20%.

Whilst exaggerated reports of longevity were gradually revised, it was possible to substantiate claims of many people to have achieved 100 years, or ages approaching that figure, when early baptismal records were found. By the early 1980s two salient factors had emerged. One was the evident fitness and mental alertness of even the oldest of the old in Vilcabamba. The second was that whilst scientists sought biological, environmental and clinical reasons for the good health of Vilcabamba residents, no attention was being paid to the quality of life at such ages.

A collaboration between the writer, the University of Loja and Dr Ken Tout produced an indepth socio-economic survey of 135 persons over 70 years of age. A surprising finding was that 96% were interested in some alternative forms of activity being set up and only 14% felt that they would not be able to take part in a novel work programme. The normal agricultural tasks were seen as excessively burdensome as a centenarian was compelled to continue the same workload as when in his or her 20s or 30s.

Migration of younger able-bodied people was becoming a problem for the remaining elderly inhabitants in Vilcabamba, as in many other developing societies. There was no desire to relinquish work entirely but simply a wish for some less onerous alternatives with additional income possibilities.

THE DEFENCE COMMITTEE

At a village meeting of 180 persons aged over 70, a 'Committee for the Defence of the Elder' was set up with the over-70s as a majority element in the committee. The elders proposed various possible initiatives to supplement or replace the normal tasks of tilling tiny corn patches located in almost inaccessible nooks and crannies of the steep hills. Health experts might consider the daily climbing and tilling to be good for longevity but the residents did not feel that such extreme activity constituted the optimum quality of life. They themselves suggested corn plots at lower altitude, poultry farming, handicrafts, tobacco growing and medicinal plant cultivation.

When land prices were taken into account, especially where flat agricultural terrain was at a premium, it proved impossible to purchase adequate land for corn or tobacco cultivation within reasonable reach of the main group of residents. A sewing room could be set up for the older women but ideas for male activity such as collecting wild grains or growing flowers offered no promise of commercial viability. In discussion with other age care organizations, it was thought that a small rural bakery could be an acceptable type of project.

Any initiative requiring an investment of cash capital would have to be funded from external sources as there was little cash movement within the valley itself. Government funds were in scant supply and the local health centre had been equipped only because of the largess of Kokichi Otani, a Japanese visitor and benefactor. Of the residents, some 65% were involved in some kind of productive activity in addition to tilling the plots of land which 53% owned, but the additional work in breeding a few domestic animals or poultry, or carrying on somewhat exotic crafts, produced only subsistence provisions and a little excess for immediate barter.

A grant was available from an international source to set up the sewing room and the rural bakery. This last consisted of primitive woodburning ovens and was located on the small central plaza. It was thought that the bakery might also double-up as a café eventually. However, it soon became apparent that the bakery could employ very few hands. The product was in no way superior to bread produced in individual homes. Local people were not accustomed to purchasing their daily bread. And the property on the plaza was a prime site which, in local terms, was expensive to rent. The sewing room, on the other hand, could pay its way eventually.

Some of the elders had originally proposed the revival and production of herbal medicines. The initial survey had also revealed that nearly 40% took a daily herbal drink and considered it to have health giving value, whilst less than 10% ever drank milk. So, as an alternative to the bakery-cum-café scheme, the herbal medicine idea was examined.

HERBAL MEDICINE GARDENS

Due to the influx and hard sell of manufactured multinational pharma-ceutical products, many of the traditional uses of herbal remedies had been forgotten. Doctors trained in the North, or trained by Northern standards, tended to deprecate the use of alternative remedies. At the same time inflation and exchange rates meant that manufactured pharmaceuticals were proving most expensive for poorer urban workers or for rural workers tied to a semi-barter system.

It would therefore be necessary for elders to share their memories of traditional remedies, both as to the type and location of the herbs and bushes involved and the precise prescription of the resultant medicines. Elders of 80, 90 and even 100 years of age played their part in a search operation to locate the various plants, berries, leaves and so on in local fields and woods, as remedies were remembered.

For the purpose of cultivation of specific herbs, a smaller space of soil was required at a much reduced cost compared with a programme of grain production. Some items could be harvested direct from the wild. But the gentle process of tending the smaller plots on level ground was much more congenial to the oldest workers than the continual trek up pre-cipitous hillsides. In this programme of remembering, searching and culti-vating, the senior was at a great advantage compared with any younger workers who might have been tempted to essay such an enterprise.

If the products from the programme were to be sold, and it was clear that these could be sold at minimal prices convenient to shoppers in poorer urban markets, then the remembered but long-forsaken remedies would need to be tested and authenticated. It therefore fell to this Director of the Health Centre, as a qualified doctor, to test the various mixtures or infusions and work out standard prescriptions for the use and safety of persons unfamiliar with these.

The sewing room presented itself as a convenient packing shop for the medicines and the elderly women there would have an additional activity in packaging doses of remedies to which a printed prescription would be attached. For both men and women there was pride in the revival of traditional 'green' methods. There was also an inflow of cash which enabled what they so much desired: a change of clothes, an addition to the normal monotonous diet or a few home comforts in the mud brick, adobe or wattle type houses in which they lived.

WELFARE 'SPIN-OFF'

Whilst the Japanese benefactor had provided funds for the health centre and there was international interest in the lack of cardiovascular illnesses in Vilcabamba, there was no global health service as such. And in the initial survey some 10% of elderly stated that they did not seek medical aid because of fears or taboos about modern medicines, 14% had indicated inability to become involved in new income generating projects and 16% suffered to some extent from mental problems. In many cases younger relatives had been lured away to the big cities in search of fortune. Only 23% lived with their families.

The Committee for the Defence of the Elder had recognized from its inception that there would be older persons who could not participate actively in the programme and some who were in dire need which the overall programme must cater for. An integral part of the first proposal was therefore the employment of a social work visitor and, in the early days, a trained nun undertook these duties. All elderly people who did not take part in the activities programme were visited in their own homes and assessed for health and social needs. Typical of the 'non-active' elders was 97 year old widow Rosa, who had no family support and no practical skills. Her daily routine was to carry her shopping bag around neighbouring houses and farms to collect donations of food. Not quite a beggar, she trudged miles daily through the hilly country. While she could walk she could eat.

A flow of aid came from a HelpAge 'Adopt a Gran' link-up but this external welfare contribution was complemented by income from local fundraising efforts as well as from profits from the income generating projects. Capital costs included much needed transport, an ambulance and a jeep, plus tools, sewing machines, initial supplies of materials and purchase of some land. It was hoped that the programme would be self-financing within two years, but a more realistic later appraisal extended this to five years.

Delays were encountered in the unsuccessful experiment with the rural bakery idea; the appointment away of an influential chairman of the Committee; the inadequacy of certain volunteers for the responsibilities of coordinating a large financial programme; the lack of 'modern' pressures which 'get things done' but which are alien to the temper and welfare of the locality; and the inevitable delays in securing international finance. The initial remembering and seeking out of medicinal plants, whilst a most valuable and prestigious contribution of the elderly themselves, was inevitably a fallow period in revenue terms. It was not considered appropriate to import an expatriate expert during the initial period as this would have been extremely costly and might have led to some cultural disagreements.

In regard to the philosophy of the programme good success may be claimed, for the Committee has always been well served by elders with a real voice in decision making, the oldest inhabitants have been offered more appropriate workloads and opportunities for earning a modest cash addition to their standard of living, those incapable of participation have been catered for, a useful local resource has been reactivated and the process has not generated any modernizing or polluting effect which might detract from the inhabitants' expectation of longer years whilst ensuring a better quality of life.

One worrying tendency has been the publicity accorded to the Valley of Long Life with the resultant initial trickle of affluent settlers from the North seeking to extend their own life expectancy in the ideal surroundings of Vilcabamba. The Government of Ecuador is sensitive to any threat to this very special group of elders and may be expected to resist any undue invasion of unwanted influences. In 1992 a new National Institute of Gerontology for Ecuador was inaugurated in Vilcabamba.

In the two year period from 1983, later extended because of delays, 'international grant aid enabled a total investment of £28 456 in the Vilcabamba programme. About a third of this was contributed in co-funding by the European Community and the major share of aid came from Help the Aged (UK). As the programme developed the total number of elderly to benefit rose to 123, including those actively participating and those receiving welfare support.

In a recent full year the total turnover of the programme was approximately £ 20 800, yielding a profit for welfare of nearly £3000. The sewing room made a profit of some £ 400. Of course, the translation of the local currency into pounds sterling fails to mirror faithfully the true impact of the scheme locally, for the equivalent of a pound sterling requires much more hard labour to produce and has much more purchasing value than the same pound sterling in the UK.

Included in the programme and budget for the year cited was a training programme initiated with Government support. This sought to make available to planners and practitioners from other parts of Ecuador the skills and experience acquired by the Committee for the Defence of the Elder. It has to be remembered that, until recent times, populations in rural Ecuador were stable and the elderly were cared for by their extended families when no longer able to cope alone. No extensive professional or volunteer care network was required. Areas such as these are only recently moving into 'age care' as a major concern. Where a programme like the Vilcabamba initiative exists it becomes the seed for wider sowing.

It is sad to record that the articulate and humorous spokesman from the first planning meeting of the Committee in 1983, 110 year old Don Manuel Ramon, died within the year before he could have full advantage of the alternative activity he craved. In his lonely hut he succumbed to an influenza attack from which he might have recovered had the health visiting programme been fully operational by then. It might be cynically questioned why a 110 year old person should desire to recover and live yet longer, adding to the world's population problems. It might be suggested, in response, that the unfrenzied, humane and useful style of survival of the Vilcabamba elders offers an alternative to the prevailing but often unsatisfying attitudes of mechanization and urbanization.

RECOMMENDATIONS

It is true that primitive people in all environments and cultures have developed their own methods of traditional medicine. With the current growth of interest in 'green' issues it is possible that groups of elders in industrialized countries also might wish to initiate a revival of their own traditional resources. Whilst in Vilcabamba such practices were recent enough to be remembered by older generations, in industrialized countries some knowledge may be totally lost to memory. A task for seniors could therefore be to research in libraries and botanical gardens, but taking care that any natural products are properly tested for safety and effect.

A particular lesson of the Vilcabamba programme is that specific programmes which involve the participation particularly of the very old may need to be paced to the requirement of that generation. In this case, a funding agency required that the project should be completed within a two year period (in order to comply with its own constitutional and mandatory regulations) but the generational reality called for something nearer a five year period of initiation. This was eventually conceded.

An allowance, both in time and capital, needs to be made for dislocation of plans where almost the entire operation depends on the work of volunteers. Force of circumstances may remove some essential personnel from the team; others may prove unskilled or not adaptable for control of vastly wider and greater issues; some may yield to the understandable temptation to compensate themselves in inappropriate ways unless strict procedures are implemented.

However, the Vilcabamba Committee does illustrate that, given true opportunities to discuss their own destinies, the oldest of the old can play a vital part in planning, conception of ideas and management decision making, rather than having to respond to decisions wholly discussed and taken by groups of younger experts.

Fuelling a small enterprise

22

An innovative Kenyan income generating scheme for elders

J. Robert Ekongot

Many elderly people are facing income problems in Kenya. Until recently the extended family system was the old person's 'pension security' but the widely acknowledged weakening of the family system, due largely to migration, has caused concern to individuals and agencies alike.

There are pensions available in Kenya but many older people, in particular in rural areas, are not eligible for them. In other cases the retirement income is not, by itself, adequate for a continued quality of living. It would be strange to suppose that, almost overnight, developing countries could set up retirement pensions or social security adequate for all needs in the way that these have evolved over a very long period in a relatively few industrialized nations (few in respect of an adequate, truly universal pension).

In addition to present concerns about family disintegration and consequent isolation of older people, Kenya, like other rapidly developing countries, is also facing a major growth of its old age population. One statistic should suffice. A United Nations forecast suggested that over the period 1980 to 2020 Kenya must expect its over-60s population to rise from about 0.5 million to nearer 3 million. If there are economic problems among older people now, what will they be in 2020 if nothing effective can be done in the interim?

Small scale income generating projects appear to be one possible response to the problem. They would have, at present, three major objectives:

1. To give immediate essential support to elders without assured means of income.

2. Marginally also to benefit the poor communities in which such older people tend to reside.
3. To act as experimental pilot models for refinement and replication against the day of much more serious problems which may accompany the greying of the nation's population.

During the 1980s HelpAge Kenya (HAK) came into being and developed into a well-known national agency with the prime aims of supporting local age care initiatives through fundraising, information and training. It was also a useful intermediary for importing significant international resources, often for projects which themselves might not have had the competence to raise funds from such sources. As time went by HelpAge Kenya became ever more involved in the detailed requirements of projects and, to facilitate this support, a Project Officer was appointed.

Already there is a range of projects which could be quoted from HAK records but the one here chosen, whilst perhaps not the most evocative, is a good example of the very low key, modest target, small group, earthy and practical idea which often gives best results, rather than some exotic idea or over-ambitious grand design.

A VISIT TO MAWEGO

Driving some five hours south west from the capital Nairobi, the visitor could arrive at the Mawego Catholic Mission in Kendu Bay, South Nyanza District of the Nyanza Province. He or she would be amazed by the numerous ongoing activities there, all aimed at improving the living standards of this rural people. Most of the activities, programmes and projects at the Mission are supervised by sisters from the order of Little Sisters of St Francis of Assisi.

The main activities to be seen include educational facilities ranging from primary through secondary levels, technical school, a bakery project, a cereal grinding mill, tailoring classes, clinic, an Adopt-a-Granny scheme and the kerosene selling project. The last two are activities meant to benefit the elderly (the one financially supported internationally, the other an income generating project). The bakery is also for the benefit of elders. In this report it is the kerosene selling programme which is featured.

In regard to elderly work, the Mission's first action was to enter and administer the Adopt-a-Granny scheme (AAG). Under this AAG system, the local agency confirms cases of very needy elderly persons who are then internationally sponsored (although first moves are already made towards effective national sponsoring) and they receive cash support on a quarterly basis.

In fact it is the caring organization which receives the cash as a block grant and thereafter distributes it as convenient to the sponsored

'Grannies'. In reality, also, both elderly men and women benefit from the AAG income and there are currently some 148 needy elders of both sexes who are registered for assistance at the Mission and who would be eligible for AAG. To date 80 of these have been found sponsorship through HAK's 'elder brother' agency, Help the Aged (UK). HAK plays the integral part of ascertaining that all information required for such sponsorship is accurate and that the aid is dispensed in the approved manner.

It was against this background of increasing numbers of elderly being identified as needing support, and the obvious logic of finding suitable local ways of developing part of the total aid, that the kerosene selling project commenced. Basically the programme was envisaged as supplementing the AAG quarterly grant to elders from the profits realized.

The coordinator of age care programmes at Mawego, Sr Mary, called a meeting of older people, both AAG sponsored and non-sponsored, not only to explain the working of the AAG scheme but to point out that local means must be sought to enhance it, both in its contribution to sponsored individuals and in taking up some of the unsponsored waiting list. The meeting was also to encourage the elders to suggest ideas as to how they might best be supported, what projects they thought could meet their needs best, in what projects they themselves might most suitably become involved and so on.

After indicating deep appreciation of what had already been achieved and expressing acknowledgement that an external scheme could not meet all their needs for ever more, the group reached a ready consensus that perhaps the most pressing material need which they all experienced at that moment was simply for kerosene (paraffin).

KEROSENE – AN ESSENTIAL ELEMENT

They explained that, as was the case with water before supplies were ensured, they had to walk, those who were able, long distances to purchase small supplies of kerosene of a quantity that they could carry back. Kerosene was a main source of light. It was also becoming more and more important as a cooking fuel because of the lack of firewood in Mawego.

In a reciprocal exchange of ideas from the elders and guidance from the sisters, the proposal emerged that a source of funding should be sought for a single substantial grant to purchase an initial large supply of kerosene for retail sale by the new project. This could be sold not only to elders but also to the general community at Mawego which had no easily accessible retail supply. It could raise some useful income for sharing among the older group. It would also be a great boon in terms of relief for sore feet, tired limbs and dispirited minds. Such was the moment of conception of the now locally famous kerosene selling project at Mawego Mission.

At this point the incipient scheme was a decision of the sisters and the elders without external advice. Sr Monica, acting on behalf of the group, contacted the familiar advice centre of HelpAge Kenya in Nairobi for assistance to work up the kerosene selling project so as to be able to interest an international source in making a grant to what might look to be a none too captivating concept.

After discussing the project with the caring organization, HelpAge Kenya conducted a survey and confirmed that a kerosene selling operation would be viable in the Mawego area. A project application was edited and financial support was received from Help the Aged (UK) AAG project. (In addition to Help the Aged's general funds, its AAG programme has its own modest but useful fund accruing from additional gifts sent in by AAG supporters and allocated to one-off projects for groups of AAG beneficiaries.)

The amount received covered all initial costs necessary to set a selling business going. Twelve drums were to serve as storage facilities for the kerosene. A kerosene pump had to be purchased. A shed was erected to house the project. The grant also covered the cost of the initial delivery of sufficient kerosene to stock the store to capacity.

Meanwhile Sister Mary, aided by the recommendations of the HAK survey and with ongoing advice from the HAK project department, began setting up the system of sales to local customers. An assistant was appointed to have day-to-day responsibility for the selling operation and other material aspects of the scheme. But little was needed in the way of advance publicity! A full bulk supply of kerosene is sold out within two weeks. Nobody is denied a supply of kerosene in cases of extreme need but generally the system works as an ordinary retailing business with active elders involved as far as possible. The catchment area of sales is about 10 kilometres square. This wide and consistent demand reveals how correct the local elders were in their anticipation of the need.

THE ESSENCE OF DEVELOPMENT

Although fully involved in consultations from an early stage, the staff of HAK were quite astonished at the profitability of this small enterprise. It has risen to a net profit of about 3000 Kenyan shillings a month, which is quite satisfying when it is realized that the total capital investment was one of the order of 43 000 Kenyan shillings, equal to about 14 months of net profit. And kerosene will be in demand locally for years to come.

It is not to be doubted that there would be problems in setting up a project for which there was no precedent, located at a fairly remote site and depending on mainly voluntary effort. In fact the greatest problem was that of spillage during the bulk delivery of kerosene. At times it was estimated that up to a full drum's capacity of kerosene had been wasted. So a plan was evolved to install an underground tank which would cause very little wastage compared with that of filling 12 separate drums. There has also been a problem with the delayed delivery of kerosene from suppliers.

If these problems can be ironed out there will be even more profit available for sharing among the local elderly. Meanwhile HAK has embarked on a two year training programme enabling all officials and care staff of all associated agencies for the elderly to study methods of achieving project efficiency. The training workshops are held at provincial level and include skills in such aspects as accounting, record keeping and leadership. The staff from Mawego attended the second of these workshops in 1991.

Project staff will continue to look for new methods of suitable income generation and to refine and adapt those methods already proven, so that the challenge of the growing population of the next decades can be met. They will have in mind that the idea for the Mawego project came from the elderly themselves. After about two years of continued success the project can truly be said to have 'fuelled' the economy of the local elderly population.

Recycling the old 23

Alternative means of income support (Colombia, India, Egypt)

Ken Tout

In their search for suitable methods of generating additional or even basic subsistence income, old people's groups have evolved a number of unusual strategies. Notable among these is the recycling programme in Pereira city, capital of Colombia's province of Riseralda.

The local Pro Vida group, under the leadership of Dr Carlos Alfonso Marin Marin, had commenced a modest programme of welfare work with the elderly but soon recognized that a priority requirement was for supplementing the meagre income which many elderly people could rely upon. A survey in Colombia at the time had revealed that only about 20% of people of retirement age had what could be regarded as a stable and sufficient source of income.

As the majority of persons eligible for pensions were employees of government or multinational concerns, they tended to reside in larger numbers in the national capital, Bogotá, and in lesser numbers in the provinces. The Pereira group therefore gave thought to the problem of the 80% who did not enjoy stable incomes, among whom were many who had no children to support them or who had been separated from their children by the forces of migration.

A DECENT AND PRODUCTIVE WAY

The recycling idea originated from a casual fusion of two observations: firstly, that many of the said 80% needed urgent means of obtaining additional income and secondly, that a number of elderly persons, in a considerable state of destitution, had been seen picking among rubbish to salvage what useful items they might be able to find. The thought evolved, 'Is there not some more decent and productive way of maximizing the use of the kind of waste which a modern city generates?'

Enquiries revealed that there was no systematic approach to redeeming those elements of rubbish which might have further use. Paper was a particular product which went, in fairly clean condition, direct to the universal burning process of the municipal rubbish collecting system. Further research proved that there did exist in Colombia a factory for recycling paper and similar materials and that it was by no means swamped with incoming materials. As a number of elderly people of certain abilities were already attending the mainly welfare and social centre of Pro Vida they were taken into the thinking and planning at an early stage.

As soon as it was agreed that a salvage project might be mounted the group realized that the same idea might occur to other less charitable forces. The local *Alcalde* (Mayor) was amenable to any initiatives which might benefit elderly persons, as well as other disadvantaged groups, so an application was made for the municipality to grant to the elders of the city the monopoly of salvage and recycling. This was readily conceded as a benevolent dispensation.

Although the elders' initiative would generate much of its own publicity through family and other community networks, it was thought that further publicity would be gained by having a uniform design of decent receptacles, rather than starting with shoddy equipment. So a special bin (*caneca*) was obtained and painted with Pro Vida colours and logo. From the commencement some 40 centres agreed to have *canecas* permanently sited on their premises, including supermarkets, offices, schools and residential blocks.

The house in which Pro Vida had its advice and social centre was built on a slope with a sizeable *bodega* underneath – a kind of small crypt. This was to serve as the store for collected materials and also a sorting base. Almost immediately it proved to be too small. The inrush of materials was so great that the Pro Vida vehicle had to be turned out of its garage in order to afford a sorting space.

The first working elders comprised three groups of four persons each, with districts allocated for collections. Elders were used at all levels of the scheme, included management, promotion, liaison with the collection points, recording and sorting in decent conditions. The public soon learned to put aside for transfer to the *canecas* clean, useful materials, with newspapers being a considerable volume of the trade. Handling this type of surplus goods was a considerable step up in prestige, sensitivity and preventive health from the previous random visits to rubbish bins.

The processing plant was able to consume all the materials which could be delivered. The growing interest, international, national and personal, in 'green' issues meant that this was an activity which was likely to gain added impetus as time went by. In addition to the paper and other textiles processed through to the factory, other donations in kind were made by the public as people became familiar with the project.

The cost of obtaining and locating the first supplies of *canecas* and of providing adequate transport was relatively high for a small non-profit group, so for the first year the project was kept to a fairly modest level with the initial three groups serving the 40 locations. This also enabled problems which might emerge to be identified, assessed and dealt with before further outlay in developing the programme. But it was then possible to justify the introduction of another 80 canecas with another 12 elderly persons lined up to join the enterprise.

Whilst this was still a low key business employing a small number of elders it had a number of significant 'spin-offs' in addition to the agreed wage which each participant was able to draw on a weekly basis. There was a useful profit which went to swell the Pro Vida welfare fund and which was specifically destined for the relief of those who would not be able to participate in any income project because of frailty or mental confusion. There was a vast increment of public interest, knowledge of ageing and goodwill towards the overall programmes. The recycling project also dovetailed into other of the Pro Vida projects.

SCHOOLS COLLABORATE

Like other Pro Vida groups, The Pereira committee had from an early period of its existence (in the late 1980s) mounted an awareness campaign in local schools. Volunteers with teaching skills visited schools to give lessons on ageing and the elderly and to encourage school pupils to become involved in intergenerational initiatives, including local fundraising. This programme had grown rapidly to embrace 33 schools and 13 000 pupils. These latter became some of the most enthusiastic protagonists of the recycling programme, acting as publicists in their families and other groups and taking part in competitions to see which school or class would collect most good salvage materials.

Income from the recycling enterprise and goodwill leading to further public financial support enabled Pro Vida to extend its general welfare programme, including a small medical and dental consulting room and other responses to perceived needs. This enabled services of one type or another to be offered to 320 elderly people of the locality who were in some kind of need of care, support or useful activity.

The elders engaged in recycling are aged between 55 to 70, as in Latin American society some underprivileged persons exhibit signs of ageing (inability to cope with normal labour tasks) from about 55 years of age or, in some places, even earlier. There is no 'retirement' limit and those participating in the programme will continue, whatever their age, whilst they are able, assured in the thought that when those tasks become too much for them they will then number among those who are in other ways benefited by the proceeds of this elders' monopoly business.

A PENSION IN FISH

An earlier initiative with similar end objectives took place in an Indian fishing village of a vastly different cultural tradition from modern Pereira city. The longer term development concept arose out of a short term desperate situation following a major natural disaster.

A cyclone which struck eastern India had devastated a considerable stretch of the coastline of Andhra Pradesh. Entire fishing villages were swept away by the storm and high tides, although the inhabitants were often able to survive by retreating inland. A typical shattered village was Pallepalem which had lost all its boats, leaving no means of continuing survival for the villagers.

As in Pereira a concept was born of two diverse considerations: on the one hand, the fisher people needed boats in order to live; on the other, the British agency Help the Aged had emergency funds available but, because of its constitution and the desires of its donors, could only contribute to a strategy which would benefit older people in a major way.

Before the cyclone the villagers had not owned their own boats, but had always had to hire them from city middlemen who charged considerable sums of money in comparison to the rather meagre income which accrued from selling surplus fish. If the fishers could own their own boats their profits would soar. The vessels used were not true watertight boats but rather boat-shaped rafts made of balsa type wood logs lashed together with ropes. The wood was not available locally, or in Andhra Pradesh at all, but had to be brought great distances from forests in Kerala.

After intense discussion it was agreed that Help the Aged would provide the cash to purchase and transport wood sufficient to construct 33 new raft-boats. Rope and new nets would also be funded. In return the villagers would form a co-operative to own the boats, three persons to each boat. From each daily catch of fish at sea, each boat would separate an agreed quantity of fish as a kind of tithe to be donated for the benefit of the elderly and younger disabled villagers who were unable to go to sea.

Some opposition was encountered initially from city businessmen who naturally wished to resume their monopoly of boat owning along that coast. They seemed intent on exerting considerable pressure of a perhaps unpleasant kind on the unsophisticated villagers of that remote fishing beach. However, the combination of Government officials and an influential international agency enabled the project to go ahead.

Given the balsa type wood and rope delivered to the beach, the local people were able quickly to construct their own traditional seagoing craft and the fishing fleet once more put out to sea. On return they found able elderly people waiting with their baskets and into these went each boat's tithe of fish. The elders were then able to sell the fish in nearby villages. As in Pereira and other similar projects, there was benefit both for the elderly salespeople, who drew a direct income, and for the most frail and disabled for whom part of the sales profit constituted a communal welfare fund.

ENHANCING THE RUBBISH JOB

Another recycling programme of a kind exists on the outskirts of Cairo, Egypt. The capital city generates thousands of tons of rubbish daily. The resultant huge rubbish heaps sustain a cultural community of about 4000 people known as the *Zabbaleen* (literally, those who live on the rubbish). The group has about 200 elderly people who must continue to work as long as they physically can as the margin of subsistence product is so small.

In this case the local charitable agency involved was not proposing any technological upgrading of the work, which would have been tremendously expensive and probably culturally disruptive. Instead they wished to concentrate on making life as bearable as possible for the elderly workers who had little access to minor comforts.

A co-funding project by the European Community and Help the Aged (UK) enabled the construction of a multipurpose centre. This was planned to a day centre model rather than as a residential institution. The elderly users were, in the main, accustomed to their simple mode of shelter and did not generally ask for an alternative. What the new building did provide was their own home-from-home where they could eat, relax, socialize and enjoy better health prospects.

Bathing facilities were an obvious priority and were warmly welcomed. Relaxation rooms were culturally furnished with low tables and cushions. A nourishing daily meal was served. Major health concerns were burns and eye disease but the centre's clinic also introduced health checks and preventive measures. The medical staff and sisters from the centre also visited frail elders in their own shelters.

Plans were laid for using part of the building as a creche for use by working mothers, where some of the able elderly women might act as childminders instead of working on the rubbish heaps. Given the restricted funding available for welfare of older people in some developing countries and especially the general lack of priority given to elder programme development in international aid systems, this type of 'health and comforts' provision for older workers, who had no cultural objection to work as such at an advanced age, was preferable to any attempt at major diversification of tasks.

CONCLUSION

Whilst somewhat ambitious in their local context, all these projects tally with the ideal requirements of an income generating scheme as detailed in Ekongot's essay on Kenya, being low key, of modest targets (by international aid standards), small group staffed, earthy and practical; of immediate benefit to the participants, but sharing some increment for the frailer and confused; and particularly susceptible to continued experimentation and replication.

PART EIGHT
Environment

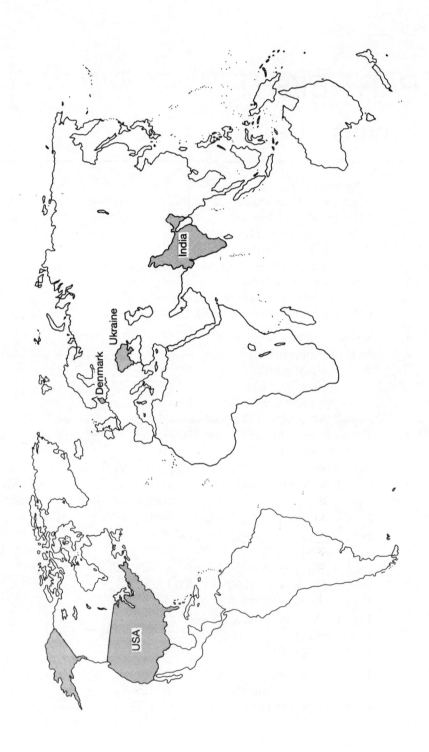

A home in Kiev 24

A special housing project for the single elderly

Vladislav V. Bezrukov, Lyudmila A. Podust and Vera V. Chaikovskaya

Ukraine is one of the oldest states within the former USSR. The number of persons 60 years and over reached 18.7% by 1989 and the average lifespan of the population is 70.9 years (66.1 for men and 75.2 for women) (Finansy, 1990). Among the consequences of demographic population ageing are significant changes in the social, economic and family status of elderly people, their health, needs for medicosocial service and care, shelter and housing.

The problem of housing and rational settling of the elderly is very acute in Ukraine. Naturally, elderly citizens have the right to decide whether they will stay with a family, live independently, at an inpatient geriatric institution or in a specialized residential home.

It should be noted that in recent times the process of disintegration of extended, multigenerational families has occurred. Increasing numbers of pensioners live separately from their adult children. In towns, up to 30% of the elderly live separately from their family members (in Kiev, up to 60%). The number of single elderly persons and ageing married couples living alone has also increased. For example, according to the data of the City Social Welfare Department, by January 1 1992 there were 15 081 persons of pensionable age registered in Kiev who lived alone. Of these, 50% needed constant social and medical care. In 1991, the population of Kiev was 2.6 million. Persons of pensionable age (males 60+, females 55+) made up 15.1% of this total.

Particularly inadequate housing conditions confront elderly persons living in the least equipped flats (without hot water, gas, telephone and other amenities), which do not meet the changing needs and physical capacities of older people. Overshadowing this is the poor infrastructure of the social and daily living services at home. All this promoted the implementation of one of the main principles of the UN International Plan of Action on Ageing – helping the aged to continue to live in their own homes and in their familiar environments for as long as possible.

The existing system of geriatric medicosocial institutions cannot meet the needs. For example, by January 1 1992, in the system of the Ministry of Social Welfare there functioned 213 nursing homes with a capacity of 46 339 places in Ukraine, including 149 nursing homes for psychogeriatric patients (33 274 places). Only a few geriatric hospitals or departments exist in the system of the Ukraine Ministry of Health.

In the early 1980s there was a special Governmental decree about construction in all large towns of special residential houses designed for single and childless pensioners, who are able to satisfy their daily domestic needs but require, at least partly, aid in daily living. By the beginning of 1988, more than 20 residential houses with a capacity of 100–300 places each had been built in the former USSR. In Kiev, the capital of Ukraine, the first such house was built in 1988.

FACILITIES OF THE KIEV HOME

The Kiev residential home is a 6-storeyed building equipped with all technical aids to meet the special needs of each tenant – enlarged doorways, wide corridors and stairs, wheelchair paths, rails in corridors, living rooms and bathrooms, an internal communication system connecting each room with an on-duty nurse, etc. It is located in the park zone in a suburb of Kiev.

It consists of 85 separate one-room flats with a bathroom, a toilet, a pantry and a kitchen to accommodate single persons and married couples. The floor area is 1147.7 sq m. On the ground floor there is a dining room, dry cleaning and laundry services, a hairdressing salon, a shoe repair shop and a library. The home has a cinema hall, a work therapy shop, an in-home workroom, a sitting room with a TV set (a sit-together place in nasty weather), a medical station and a physiotherapist's room.

STAFF AND MEDICAL SERVICES

The total number of staff is 30 persons, including administrator, manager, accountants, medical personnel (two physicians and five nurses), social workers, etc.

The medical aid is provided by a therapist and a neuropathologist, both part-time staff, five nurses and four nurse assistants. The medical station works throughout 24 hours and has an internal communication with every living unit. In addition, the necessary outpatient medical aid for the tenants is made available by one of the district polyclinics. Periodically, medical consultations are given by the professionals of the Kiev Institute of Gerontology. Inpatient services are provided by town clinical hospital no. 26 and the Institute of Gerontology.

RESIDENTS

In October 1992 there were 83 persons living in the home, including 67 single elderly persons and eight married ageing couples. The average age of tenants was 75 years (men 72, women 76 years). The age–sex structure of the home residents is as follows: persons aged 75 years and over make up 43% and the ratio of men to women is 1:4 (16 males and 67 females).

Resettling to the home may take place provided the ageing person is self-sufficient and gives his or her State-owned flat to the State. Before moving to the home, the elders lived alone and had neither children nor close relatives in this town. As the main reason for their decision to resettle in the home, they mention an increasing need for medicosocial services in view of worsening health, restricted mobility and self-service abilities. Of paramount importance in decision making is the fact that on moving into the home the elderly persons will need to make virtually no essential changes to their mode of life because there will be no need for them to break an established life stereotype of behaviour. They will have favourable conditions to maintain their autonomy and former friendly contacts, as well as to establish new interpersonal relationships.

HEALTH STATUS

As in all aged populations, the tenants of the home suffer from complex and multiple pathology. The predominant kinds of pathology include ischaemic heart disease, hypertensive disease, bone and joint diseases, nervous system and sense organ diseases. There is a high prevalence of chronic diseases in compensated (47%) and decompensated (54%) forms. Among the residents, 23% are unable to serve themselves and they are taken care of by two social workers, and 11% are in need of daily medical input from paramedicals and physicians who are allocated to receive patients within home premises.

During 1989–1992, annually some 30–70% of all residents were hospitalized because of exacerbation of diseases, requiring treatment in hospital conditions. As a rule, after 3–4 weeks' treatment, these patients return to their flats in the residential home. Death rate of home residents was 1% in 1989, 2% in 1990, 4% in 1991 and 2% in 1992.

To monitor the health level and functional state of elderly persons and to assess their needs in various types of institutional/non-institutional care, at the Institute of Gerontology an automated system of quantifying the dependency of elderly persons on outside assistance has been devised (Bezrukov *et al.*, 1991). This method both evaluates the state of separate organ systems, physical and psychological status and estimates the integral index of a person's dependency on outside assistance, and needs in various kinds of medicosocial service (residential house, nursing home, hospital for long term stay).

With the use of this system, the analysis of health and self-service abilities of residents of the home during four years (1989–1992) was made. The findings showed that there were mistakes at the first stage when the tenants were settled in this home which made the work of the personnel difficult. In 1988, 13% of all residents needed to be placed in nursing homes and 3% in hospitals for the chronically ill. By 1992, these figures increased to 23% and 17%, respectively. In other words, large percentages of residents were misplaced and their needs for constant, extensive medical aid and care were unmet. They did not fit the place conditions and personnel potentialities.

Based on the results of the complex medical examination and following the recommendations of the Institute of Gerontology, in the summer of 1992 15% of residents were transferred to a newly opened nursing home.

MEALS

During first three to three and a half years, the majority of residents cooked their own meals in their flats. Only 25–30% of them used to have their lunch in the common dining room, where meals were provided for moderate fees by the staff. However, with increasing prices of food products, the pension appeared to be not enough to buy either foodstuffs or meals in the dining room. Then the town social welfare department made an additional payment to each tenant and now practically all home residents have their meals in the dining room.

PAYMENTS

The costs necessary for construction and maintenance of the home are covered by the State. All daily living and communal services are paid for by the residents themselves at a reduced price. The residents are eligible for all types of income (pensions, any other earnings).

The residents may want to conclude an agreement with the social worker to perform various kinds of work, like cleaning windows and floors, laundering, cooking food, etc. For residents with restricted mobility and significantly reduced or lost self-service abilities, all services are provided free of charge. The able residents receive an additional payment for work participation.

MODE OF LIFE

The majority of the residents lead a passive and secluded mode of life. When asked to complete a questionnaire, 80% of them reported no wish to engage themselves in any social activity or to attend work therapy shops or clubs, the main reason being poor health. However, 14% of the residents participate in the choir and there are small plots near the home for those who like to grow flowers and vegetables. Concerts, lectures and visiting of theatres and museums are regularly arranged.

CONCLUSIONS

In this country, the construction of special residential homes provided with a complex of social, daily living and medical services seems to be a prospective (though not ultimate) way of solving the problem of housing for lonely elderly persons with mild to moderate loss of capacities.

Provision is being made for adaptation of homes to accord with the needs and physical capacities of older persons. Conditions are created to provide different levels of social and daily living services. Efforts are made to bring the primary medical care closer to the elderly. Psychological and other kinds of support are also envisaged.

At the same time, these homes are being built far from the former places of elderly people's residence. This results in the breaking of previous relations, losing of habitual contacts and difficulties in adaptation to new surroundings.

The concentration in such homes of elderly persons, each one having his or her own life concept, views and habits, creates predisposition for conflicts. In this context, the roles of a psychologist and a psychotherapist become especially important. Yet these specialists are rarely included in the staff of these homes.

A serious problem is the loss of ability for self-service due to disease or trauma. The sociomedical staff allocated to the home are not sufficient. There appears to be the need for an institutionalization into nursing homes or hospitals for chronically ill patients and this may lead to new hardships.

However, the economic crisis sweeping the country impedes the development of this form of aid to the elderly. The spiral of hyper-inflation and shortage of municipal means has decelerated the process of realization of the plans to build in Kiev six more homes of this type, thus aggravating even further the existing difficulties. Progress towards solution of this question is feasible only with the normalization of the State's economy and also by seeking support from the emerging private businesses.

Simply, the best housing

25

Special housing for elders in India and similar societies

Dalip L. Kohli

The housing needs of the elderly in India have to be gauged from existing and perspective housing shortages in the context of India's population growth, the figures of population of the elderly (60+) over the decades and the expected growth hereafter, as also in the context of the rapidly growing urbanization and growth of slums in urban areas.

The housing shortage, which was reckoned at 23.3 million units in 1981, is expected to grow to 41 million units in 2001. The population of the elderly in India was 12 million in 1921, 20 million in 1951, 43 million in 1981 and the projection for 2000 is 76 million. Coming to urbanization, India's metropolitan towns have increased from five in 1951 to 12 in 1981 and 23 in 1991. Urban population, which was 11% of the total in 1901, was 25% in 1991 and is expected to reach 330 million in 2001. An estimated 30% of the population in metropolitan cities live in slums and squatter settlements; 50% of the population in Bombay and 45% in Delhi is living in such settlements. Total slum population is expected to reach 62 million by 2000, of which 32 million would be living in metropolitan cities.

These statistics will give some idea of the housing problems faced by the elderly, particularly those who are in urban areas. They are among the weakest elements and are suffering the most. Strains on the continuance of the joint family, because of inflation and urbanization and change in lifestyles of the younger members who migrate in search of livelihood, have left the elderly in a difficult situation. Where they are able to accompany their children to urban areas, they are marginalized because of overall housing shortages. Taking up of careers by daughters and daughters-in-law has taken away the care and comfort which the elderly have obtained in the past for their needs.

A DESIGN FOR LIVING

With the staggering shortages and rising costs housing for the elderly has to be provided by families concerned or by voluntary organizations, in the absence of any real social security programme by the Central and State Governments. The cost has to be kept down consistent with the minimum needs of the elderly. Some time ago, HelpAge India commissioned a famous architect, Laurie Baker, a naturalized Indian who has over the decades experimented extensively with local materials and with housing designs suitable for Indian climatic conditions, to make traditional living possible at low cost. Mr Laurie Baker produced an action paper with actual drawings to show what was possible and desirable for the housing needs of the elderly in India.

HelpAge India, in collaboration with HelpAge International (whose Special Representative I was for the International Year of Shelter for the Homeless, 1987) produced a publication, *Architectural Design for Housing the Elderly*, which was presented at the meeting of the United Nations Commission on Shelter for the Homeless, held at Nairobi in 1987. A reference to the publication will give fuller information on the designs. The factors which have to be kept in view are indicated below.

MATERIAL

Although cleanliness and efficiency are required when looking after old people, they are mainly not happy and do not feel at home in so-called 'modern' surroundings, with a preponderance of glass and concrete and steel. They belong to a generation which appreciated the 'natural', simple, direct building materials such as wood, mud, tile, thatch and brick. 'Contemporary' and 'modern' research has been done so that the shortcomings of these 'oldfashioned' materials have been removed and coped with. These new techniques with old materials are undoubtedly less expensive than currently fashionable materials such as cement and steel. It must be kept in mind that India will remain short of cement for quite a long time. It is an essential item for engineering work, but we have effective alternatives for domestic building work so it is necessary to use cement sparingly.

Lime is an older and well-tried material for mortars and plasters. It is as good as cement if pozzolanas (volcanic ash based) are added. A one part lime, two parts Surki, (pozzolana) four parts sand formula gives a first class mortar. In many districts mud mortars have been used effectively for centuries. There is no need to rule this out.

SPECIFICATIONS

Mud walls have been in use for centuries and are excellent when stabilized with lime or bitumen or reinforced with bamboo, husks, etc. The use of a simple, removable, adjustable frame into which earth is rammed can eliminate that 'oldfashioned' look and give a strong loadbearing wall.

Burnt brickwork is increasing in cost but a 25% reduction of bricks and mortar is effected if 'rat-trap' bond is used. It also provides better insulation and is strong and loadbearing.

The use of plaster accounts for about 10% of the total cost of a house. Furthermore, one gets committed to decoration and maintenance costs for ever more! In most districts, if a roof overhang is provided, plaster is totally unnecessary on the exterior walls of a building. Internally, if colour or whitewash is required (again, not strictly necessary) it can be applied equally well to flushpointed smooth brick work. So, we don't need to use plaster unnecessarily.

Lintels are usually overdesigned or even totally unnecessary. Use simple lintels or use reinforced brick. Save cement, save steel, save cost.

Timber is now costly. Consider using treated 'country timbers' and use minimum sections ($2\frac{1}{2}" \times 3\frac{1}{2}"$ is adequate for door and window frames.)

The oldfashioned floor tile or 'brick tile' or 'quarry tile' is comfortable, homely and 'good for rheumatism'. These tiles are far superior, for old people, to mosaic, terrazzo and polished stone. All forms of cement flooring are found to be 'cold' and they 'sweat' badly during the monsoon.

In districts where it is available and suitable, use should be made of tiled roofing rather than reinforced concrete. Where reinforced concrete is considered essential, then make a 30% reduction in cost and in cement by using a filler slab or a ribbed slab or any of the cement and cost-reducing systems developed by the CBRI (Central Building Research Institute) at Roorkee, UP, India. Similarly for economical use of wood, consult the Forest Research Institute of Dehra Dun.

Where glazed tiles are desirable but too costly, use the cheapest form of glass (ribbed or reeded glass is best) cut into large tile shapes and use on walls exactly as you use tiles. This gives a washable smooth surface which is as strong as tile and a quarter the cost. (Be sure to eliminate air bubbles from behind the glass tiles!)

In many districts throughout India, black cotton soil poses foundation problems. Do not waste money on excessive excavations and infillings, or on piles or reinforced concrete rafts. For buildings of the type suitable for the elderly, surface beams of large aggregate concrete make a combined foundation-cum-plinth and prevent future wall cracks. Reinforcement can be of bamboo where good mature bamboo is available.

Do not use ground or milk glass in windows. Old people like to see what is going on outside.

DESIGN

For the convenience of the elderly, some of the suggestions made by Laurie Baker are as follows:

- Avoid double storey buildings. Avoid all steps and stairs. If different levels are unavoidable, use gentle ramps. Don't forget that this includes the difference between outside ground level and inside floor level.

- Things for daily use should be stored at heights between 2' and 6' only. Only seasonal storage (such as winter clothes and blankets) may be stored low down (such as in drawers under the bed).
- Where stooping is unavoidable (squatting on an Indian-type latrine), provide strong handles so that one can pull oneself up again.
- Avoid low-down storage places in kitchens. After 60, backs no longer bend easily. Getting back to an upright position is even more difficult.
- Strong handles or rails fixed on to walls near seats and beds are greatly appreciated.
- Avoid slippery, shiny, overpolished floors and use non-slip or non-skid surfaces to ramps, kitchen and bathroom floors, etc.
- Don't forget to give a non-slip surface to the ramp from the garden up to the entrance.
- Make doors wide enough (3' 9") for two people to get through side by side. Wheelchairs may have to be used (including and especially bathroom doors).
- Provide good natural and artificial lighting. Put switches and handles where they can easily be seen. Old folk need good natural and artificial light, simple, neat, convenient furniture with storage spaces, and all within easy reach from the bed. Solid built-in furniture costs very little more than the flooring which would have been necessary if the furniture had not been 'built-in'.
- Simple colour wash on exposed unplastered brick work, with a few flowers and pictures, make a place homely and friendly.
- Provide reachable, easy catches, locks and fasteners.

HOUSING UNITS

Apart from conveniences within, Laurie Baker has given designs for single-room cottages along with bathroom and kitchenette and a small space to sit out in the shade. While elderly people appreciate privacy, by combining two, three and one-room units, a feeling of security can be given to the older residents. Ward-type dormitories have been designed with sitting and dining space. Ward-type cottages have also been designed which are better and more homely.

CLIMATIC REQUIREMENTS

While the suggestions and designs of Laurie Baker are related to the people and conditions obtaining in India, considering that India comprises several climatic zones ranging from tropical, subtropical, dry arid to cold and mountainous regions, there is a plethora of materials and designs traditional in the different climatic zones which can be adapted for use in other countries as well. The National Buildings

Organization of the Government of India has researched into traditional materials and designs and has also devised improvements which make use of traditional materials more lasting and aesthetically pleasing.

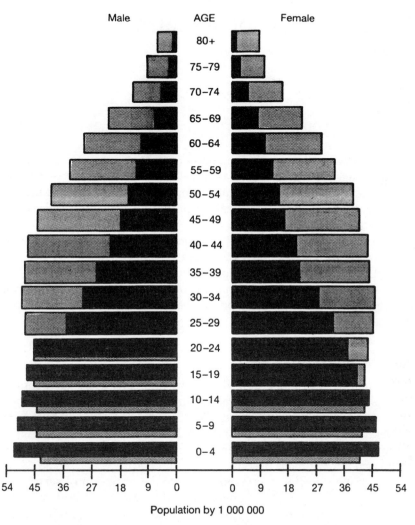

Typical 'ageing' country: Less children/ever increasing older groups

International Institute on Ageing (United Nations, Malta) age composition projects for India (1990 – dark, 2025 – light) (from Garrett, 1992)

Congregate housing 26

The multifunctional centre – the Danish experience

George W. Leeson

DaneAge (EGV) is a non-profit making organization founded in 1910 by a Copenhagen clergyman. It has developed in the course of 80 years form a local 100% voluntary organization providing shelter and meals to a national, professional organization providing housing, services, consultancy, etc. for elderly people.

The objective of DaneAge in its profound simplicity is to 'help' elderly persons. This objective entails a very broad contact with elderly in a wide field of activities and the provision of suitable housing and service, clubs, travel, activities, etc. Much is done in co-operation with local authorities and much is done on a purely private basis, e.g. travel activities, activity centres.

THE DANISH SITUATION

In Denmark, service, specialized housing and care of elderly people as well as social services in general are financed almost entirely by taxes and managed by local authorities. We have around 270 local authorities in Denmark, most of them with 5000–20 000 inhabitants. DaneAge, in conjunction with the agency Senior Tjenesten a.s., works together with about one third of these in some way or another.

The local authorities are responsible for the provision of services for the elderly and it is therefore only natural that DaneAge co-operates very closely with these authorities, both with regard to building and operational activities but also as strategic planning consultants. As far as residential nursing homes and specialized housing are concerned, co-operation with local authorities is an absolute must. Other types of housing for elderly are also built with a lesser degree of close co-operation.

The residential nursing home in its hitherto institutional form is a thing of the past. Certainly in Denmark, recent legislation means that no more residential nursing homes will be built. Residential nursing homes have a strong institutional character – smallish flats, a concentration of elderly people in need of fairly extensive care, a closed environment – and the nursing home is often far removed from the requirements made to suitable modern housing for elderly people. Only a very small minority, 5% of elderly people, live in such homes.

With the gradual disappearance of residential nursing homes, the intention is that elderly people in need of fairly extensive care should be offered a move to small scale congregate housing projects, providing them with their own independent homes in contact with people not necessarily in need of the same degree of extensive care, both younger and older, and in proximity of care and services as required and as individually assessed. Such a move stimulates their self-help capacities, improves their powers of self-determination and increases their status of equality.

CONGREGATE HOUSING

So-called congregate housing is to all intents and purposes ordinary housing, where the individual dwelling comprises two rooms in addition to a kitchen, bathroom, toilet and hall. Congregate housing contains facilities for handicapped persons, so that individual residents are able to cope on their own, even if they are in a wheelchair. There are emergency response systems by which help can be called to the individual dwelling in an emergency situation at any time of the day via a service and care centre. There is access to common rooms, where a variety of activities, service and contact are all available. Congregate housing developments ideally comprise 12–20 houses on one site. In a well-defined geographical area it is then possible to have a number of such developments with a common service centre, which could in fact be located in the local nursing home if it is still in use. These small developments are then under the jurisdiction of the local home help and district nursing which are also based in the centre, thereby ensuring continuity moving from the 'community' to the scheme. In all developments, service and assistance are flexible, provided only in accordance with self-help principles based on individual assessment and the real need.

A move into congregate housing is not necessarily conditional on a need for service. Therefore, it is possible when letting such housing units to ensure a suitable mixture of residents according to needs – the more resourceful then being able to encourage and help the less fortunate.

Experience with such congregate housing projects is extremely positive. The provision of service only as required (and not in the form of a 'package deal') – in accordance with self-help principles – together with the on-hand help and indeed the general atmosphere means that elderly persons are able to remain in such housing projects even when rather extensive service is required. Transfers to residential nursing homes are kept to an absolute minimum.

The central service centre is in daily contact with all residents unless they have specifically stated that they do not want this service. Attendant nursing staff provide individual care when required and attend to the elderly in case of acute illness. Hospitalization is also kept to an absolute minimum.

DaneAge regards this type of combined housing/service/activity scheme as the basic model for the future, but with scope for variations, so that special activities and the like can be incorporated as required, e.g. self-governing clubs, day centres, day homes, housing for other age groups, intergenerational activities, kindergartens, etc., as we shall describe later in the specific case of Æblehaven.

DEVELOPING A SCHEME

Before developing a scheme, DaneAge carries out a complete analysis of the existing local facilities for the provision of service for elderly in co-operation with the relevant professional groups in the area. A study is made of population development, residents in homes, suitable housing potential, health status, home help, meals on wheels, etc.

An interview study can also be carried out among the future elderly (50–64 years) to determine their expectations, wishes, demands for old age in the particular municipality. It is also important to elucidate actually what resources the inhabitants themselves have that could perhaps be better exploited to their own and the community's benefit.

Information briefings are held with local authority staff, existing residents/consumers and local pensioners' associations. Local press coverage is ensured in order to inform the general public of the projects/studies. The project becomes very much a community affair from the beginning.

The analysis concludes with strategic planning models designed to provide the local authority with a plan to develop their provision of service/housing/activities for the elderly.

When it has been decided to start such a scheme, a local non-profit, self-governing institution is established. DaneAge may be represented in this local institution along with local authority and professional representatives. At a later stage, staff and users are also represented on the governing body that is responsible for the day-to-day running of the centre and its economy.

As a private organization, DaneAge has to supply a product to the authorities which is better and cheaper than other available products and at the same time it must be ensured that the basic objectives of the organization are met and its philosophies pursued. This requires a continual process of development and very great efforts on the part of staff, the aim being to constantly influence attitudes and to offer a good supply of relevant training courses. These efforts are directed towards users, local civil servants and politicians, volunteers and salaried staff, not to mention the public at large.

In view of the democratic principles governing all decision making processes in modern society, it is only natural that the governing body of each centre guarantees all groups concerned representation. The individual centres have a governing body which is legally and financially responsible for running operations. Committees may be set up, as required, to look after all kinds of activities within the range of objectives of the centre in question. Moreover, the councils have a very important function as a means of communication between the governing body and the 'grass roots'.

A TYPICAL MULTIFUNCTIONAL CENTRE

The typical local authority area to be considered has a population of approximately 12 000, with 2000 persons aged 65 years and over. The annual local authority budget for elderly services would be a total of £17 800 000 breaking down into:

- Social pensions   £11 000 000
- Nursing homes   £3 500 000
- District nurses   £250 000
- Home help   £1 000 000
- Rental allowances   £800 000
- Transport, etc.   £1 250 000

The centre in question administers a total of 57 dwellings, seven of which are in a modernized and refurbished residential nursing home. These dwellings are distributed in three groups throughout the municipality.

The dwellings are furnished according to the resident's individual needs and also meet the demands for people in wheelchairs. Should a resident need immediate help there is a round-the-clock alarm system in each dwelling linked either to the centre's own alarm switchboard or the local emergency services. The size of each dwelling is 60 square metres with a small garden of five square metres and a shed. There is a kitchen, a sitting room, a bedroom and a toilet/bathroom. The average age of the residents is 78 years.

A typical centre is based on the Health Department of the Æblehaven municipality.

- The home help and district nurse have their base here. They offer their help to the centre's residents but also to other elderly persons in the community;
- There is a kitchen producing 200 meals daily, of which 150 portions are distributed to elderly living in their own homes;
- There is physiotherapist, a chiropodist and a hairdresser. These services are available to anyone, not only the elderly;
- The Activity Centre itself is designed in accordance with a large open plan with workshop facilities, a sitting room, a dining room, a cafeteria, lecture rooms for courses of all kinds and facilities for private parties, etc.

The average number of day guests is 60. Furthermore, there are ten day home guests needing special care and services – some being transported in wheelchairs.

The staff comprises 15 fulltime employees, seven volunteers and one driver who delivers the meals to the elderly in the community and transports 25 persons to and from the centre every day. All activities provided are the results of co-operation between the residents in the dwellings linked to the centre and the daily visitors.

Activities available include:

- Cafeteria   – open for all visitors
- China painting   – 2 classes
- Painting, sewing and knitting   – every day
- Courses in foreign languages   – 2 classes
- Theatre   – frequently
- Billiards   – every day
- Song classes   – 1 class
- Entertainment in evenings   – once a month;
- Pottery   – 1 class = 8 persons
- Lectures about tours and various artists – twice a month
- Folk dance   – 40 persons every week
- Gymnastics   – 2 classes
- Cooking   – 2 classes
- Bingo   – twice a month
- Physiotherapy   – open for all visitors
- Hairdresser   – open for all visitors
- Chiropodist   – open for all visitors

Other facilities are a stone grinding machine, weekend open functions, bridge, private parties, day trips, courses in the law of succession, films, weekly group meetings with elderly blind persons, society clubs and associations.

The economy of the centre is as follows:

Prices per day:

Daily visit incl. coffee and transport	£1.00
Day home incl. 3 meals, coffee and transport	£3.00
One portion 'meals on wheels'	£2.40
Dinner in the cafeteria for the elderly	£2.40
Dinner in the cafeteria for guests	£4.00
Total expenses per annum	£750 000

Annual income:

Meals on wheels	£100 000
Users' payments	£14 500
Cafeteria sale, parties, etc.	£33 500
Rent from the Health Department	£17 000
Rent from hairdresser, chiropodist	£5 000
Total income	£170 000
The municipality's annual expenses	£580 000

Elder villages: ghettos or godsends? 27

Buying into a new community to age well through 'affinity bonding' in the USA

Otto von Mering and Sharon Gordon

In the USA, a country without a universal health care system, access to available and needed services has become less certain during the past two decades and unaffordable for an extended period of illness (*Consumer Reports*, 1992). The spectre of becoming a medicated welfare statistic in a nursing home has become a reality for many. It is felt by people of all ages and expressed freely among the low and middle income segments of society. A forbidding scenario of post-retirement existence is documented in a 1991 issue of *Consumer Reports*:

> Some Americans pay all [the cost of nursing home or at home health care] with money saved. Others start paying with savings, then turn to Medicaid when they become 'medical indigents'. Still others use Medicaid from the start, and a few will use a so-called 'medigap' insurance policy.
>
> (*Consumer Reports, 1991, p. 425, 429*)

> The insurance industry is urging long-term care policies on consumers, and government officials are eager to cut the Medicaid budget. The policies themselves, though somewhat improved since 1988, still have significant shortcomings: tricky provisions in the way they are written; the potential for large rate increases; uncertainty about whether claims will be paid; and confounding policy language.
>
> (*Consumer Reports, 1991, p. 425*)

And, according to US Census Bureau data, 'The number of Americans without health insurance rose to 35.4 million in 1992, the greatest **total** since introduction of Medicare and Medicare programs in the 1960s'.

LIFE-CARE COMMUNITIES

Since the early 1970s, a rising number of people of middle income means, at the time of early or normal retirement and especially during their 70+ years, have used their disposable income to live out their lives in planned, self-governed and financed retirement communities. Most of these full-service communities, ranging in size from 250 to 750 members, are comparable to small villages and located near small towns in a rural setting. A small, but growing number are near urban centres, in a standard metropolitan statistical area, with as many as 1000 to 2500 residents.

These 'life-care' oriented communities strive to be secure residential environments which optimize shared life experience and activities among like-minded people. As such, they are intended to provide optimum opportunity for independence as residents age. As physical and mental functions become less manageable for residents, these villages assure a familiar living environment with quick and sustained access to graduated and mixed levels of personal health care and supportive service on an individual basis (Tilson, 1990).

During the past two decades, this kind of planned elder village has come to be known as a Continuum of Care Retirement Community (CCRC). CCRCs are not new not-for-profit social and residential inventions; they have existed for 100 years in the USA (Somers and Spears, 1992). According to the American Association of Homes for the Aging (AAHA), a CCRC is defined as a habitat:

> that offers a full range of housing, residential services and health care in order to serve its older residents as their needs change over time. This continuum consists of housing where residents live independently and receive certain residential services such as meals, activities, housekeeping and maintenance; support services for disabled residents who require assistance with activities of daily living (ADL); and health care service of those who become temporarily ill or who require long-term care.

Regardless of their size, great differences in the quality of extended assisted living and health services exist among CCRCs. However, the majority, in addition to offering 24-hour nursing home care, try to provide at least two general types of residential support services, one for the physically 'frailing' but mentally alert individuals and the other for the mentally 'fraying' person who is physically able. The former group of residents experience increasingly debilitating conditions like arthritis, hypertension and diabetes, as well as problems with ADL, requiring some assistance with bathing, toileting, grooming, ambulation, eating and/or medication. The latter group includes people who have exhibited dementing behaviour including rising difficulty in comprehending the environment, becoming more easily confused or lost in a familiar setting and eventually showing irretrievable restlessness, irritability and problematic conduct.

The most sophisticated of these villages function as 'total communities' which have succeeded in creating many layers of residential treatment environments so their nursing facility has come to be viewed only as a 'sub-acute hospital' where only the most impaired residents are domiciled. This layering and mixing of different individual case indicated treatments is made possible by an on-site, comprehensive home care programme. It ranges from homemaker and IADL services (e.g. cleaning and personal assistance in going to the doctor or grocery shopping) to post-hospital recuperative health care, as well as continuous or intermittent on-site clinical service visits by skilled physical therapists, occupational therapists, respiratory therapists and nurse practitioners.

A 1990 *Consumer Report* estimates that presently about 800 CCRCs are the residencies of over 230 000 elderly in the USA. It has been projected that as many as 1500 CCRCs will be the domicile of 450 000 residents toward the end of this decade. An optimistic scenario that CCRCs may be affordable for up to 50% of USA elderly has also been painted and some economists have predicted that 18.25% of people aged 75 and over will reside in CCRCs by the year 2020 (Rivlin and Wiener, 1988).

It is granted that when given a choice, older people assess their needs realistically and choose an environment that has the best probability of meeting their needs. This gerontological dictum seems underpinned by the idea that it is preferable to thrive with enterprise in a new habitat than to drift into terminal debility where you are now (von Mering, 1992a). A well-managed CCRC with age-sensitive interpersonal public and domestic spaces of caring and community activity may well be a comforting answer for someone who is considering a new life chapter with new neighbours.

THE LAKEVIEW TERRACE CCRC

It is best to examine these issues more closely in light of a community which we have studied intermittently since 1985. It goes by the name of Lakeview Terrace Retirement Community and is located on a 210 acre tract of rural land in central Forida, not far from a mid-sized town with several hospitals and assorted group practice clinics.

Since its establishment in 1975, Lakeview has been among the first Florida CCRCs with three distinct health care related state licences: home health, skilled nursing/convalescent care and adult 'semi-independent' congregate living. Independent living residual units include the standard personal amenities and food and recreational fitness services characteristic of contemporary hotels. The health care facility contains private or semi-private units that accommodate the individual needs of the resident. The community as a whole is certified by the State Insurance Commissioner as a fully qualified life-care endowment or lease option, each with a monthly service charge.

Various sized apartments and maisonettes are available within a fee schedule, ranging from the 'lowest endowment' of $29 500 with a monthly service charge (MSC) of $540 to the 'highest endowment' of $70 000 with a monthly service charge of $1320. In the course of finalizing an 'occupancy agreement', an income to monthly fee ratio formula is used to determine adequate income. The resident marketing adviser does not reveal the average income of the residents. However, he is secure in stating that for a couple, annual income begins at around $25 000.

As a part of joining the village community, newcomers are expected to join the Lakeview Terrace Residents' Association, Inc. Its bye-laws stress fundraising and the promotion of 'beneficent co-operation' between residents and management. There is a Board of Directors consisting of a president, president-elect, secretary, treasurer and two resident representatives at large. This board is also referred to as the executive committee and meets with the manager of operations the first Wednesday of every month. These meetings seem beneficial to both residents and staff not only for problem solving, but also timely intervention to avert the possible need for crisis management. Residents are frequently recognized for bringing wisdom and common sense to seemingly complicated issues.

Certain key community activities are reflected in the following standing committees of the Residents' Association: (1) welcome to new residents; (2) remembrance; (3) special projects; (4) community store; and (5) activity calendar. The agendas are prepared for the community as a whole and the health care centre complex with the help of staff. Both agendas are open to **all** residents and the residents' choices and involvement usually reflect their physical, mental and emotional abilities. The residents have a great deal of input in the design of the activities programme. Moreover, surveys are conducted every other year and input occurs through daily interaction with residents.

The Lakeview Community has remained a small face-to-face village, with a population mix favourable to diverse and multilayered ways of living. A quick summary of current statistics (May 1992) on the community, the health care enterprise and overall staffing indicates that a current population of 258 (of whom 184 are women and with an overall average age of 82) is served by a staff of about 70 nurses, assistants, home health aides and resident companions.

The most notable point is the ratio of total residents to those occupying an intensive care bed. Out of a total of 258 residents only 20 are currently occupying a nursing home bed (7.75%). This unusually low proportion of 24-hour care clients in a CCRC with an average age of 82 years can be explained in a large measure by certain distinct features of ageing in place in Lakeview.

Unlike many CCRCs, Lakeview Terrace does not operate under the traditional 'downhill all the way' view of old age. Instead, it relies on a 'terminal drop' model of ageing which corresponds to the postulate of 'rectangularization of mortality' and 'compression of morbidity' (Wilson, 1991). Lakeview Terrace has a policy perspective which stresses 'life as a continuing process' (Riker, 1990) and that lifelong learning is not just an option but a social commitment. Moreover, Lakeview seeks to optimize special health promotion, convalescent and rehabilitative services for every resident on an as-needed basis in light of changing health conditions. No one is simply 'discharged' from an assisted living environment, for example, to the intensive 24-hour nursing care unit. Whenever feasible, all residents are expected to return to their previous level of functioning. This approach abates the fears of premature frailty, loss of self-esteem and lack of independence which could otherwise weigh heavily upon many residents.

Perhaps there are some even more important reasons why Lakeview has not become just another residential retailer of graduated wellness care and 24-hour nursing services. Over the years, Lakeview appears to have developed an enduring, comforting interplay of formal and informal 'caring for' and 'caring about' its residents. Parenthetically speaking, labour turnover among key staff has been negligible over a ten-year period. That is to say, everyone seems to have learned to bestow 'social significance' to the interdependent relationship between caregivers, whether formally structured and prepaid or informally arranged among residents and staff. Residents involve themselves in progressive volunteerism, deploying their talent and lifelong skills in an effective community-wide manner.

Thus, formal care which rests on a formal knowledge base, in which professionals are trained and acquire particular skills, complements the knowledge of informal care which is rooted in daily experience and assumed to be open to all. This knowledge of persons and locality intertwines with formal caregiver knowledge for the benefit of every resident. This special co-mingling of formal and informal care, the latter being performed by volunteers among the residents, succeeds in blurring the odious Medicare payment eligibility distinction between being a 'homebound' and 'non-homebound' person when requiring assistance from another person or an assistive device.

THE AFFINITY BONDING PRINCIPLE

The community capitalizes from the very beginning on a characteristic of human life important to all people. It is the formation and reinforcing of a sense of personal affinity between residents in light of who they think they are, how they fit into their environment and how they developed comparable aspirations and shared motivations. The relevance of 'affinity groups' (Moore, 1992) in market segmentation for resident recruitment is recognized among astute developers and promoters of retirement communities. However, it is still insufficiently appreciated among many as a special resource and opportunity for creative, cost-effective and continuous caring into the last year of life. Further explanation is needed to understand how important it has been for Lakeview Terrace.

In essence, Lakeview Terrace evolved a well-balanced reliance on recruiting and retaining prospective residents who are drawn from natural affinity groups, both outside and inside Florida. These are persons who during their middle adult and pre-retirement years 'aged in place' in geographically identifiable neighbourhoods. Moreover, in their accustomed prior habitat, they shared certain social, educational, denominational, work and leisure activity bonds, typical of their generational membership in a given ethnic group, in this case WASP, or white, Anglo-Saxon, protestant. That is to say, Lakeview Terrace residents are people who bring with them a public and private world seen through similar sights and sounds, feelings and experiences, and distinct ways of caring for oneself and caring for others. They are inclined to identify with certain personal time-frames of music, socio-political issues, economic and military events of a given historical era. In short, they interpret the 'now' of their personal lives and of current events in light of these perspective.

We are proposing that the success of a CCRC over the long run actually derives from a classic conceptualization of group processes. We call it the 'affinity bonded group' principle. It is the natural social process of forming a multifaceted, face-to-face association and behavioural tendencies among people who have been living in comparable geographically defined places of residence during their adult, pre-retirement years. In so doing, these persons have become accustomed to rely on characteristic patterns of separateness from, affiliation with and support of each other. They also learned to practise analogous ways of fellowship with or aloofness from the rest of the world.

An affinity bonded group is a state of existence as much as a place. It speaks of a sense of special attachments and belonging that gives people with a particular lifestyle the confidence to prevail over changes to find the best way of adapting to their environment. A retirement community like Lakeview Terrace seeks to re-invent the opportunity for every resident to become part of such a familiar social group dynamic. It replicates and expands on the residents' preferred life ways, working careers and habits associated with their former long term places of residence. It makes ageing in place personally and socially acceptable without depleting financial assets as long term care needs increase. Above all, being a member of an affinity bonded group makes it possible to keep one's dependency on others a private rather than public matter.

It can be said that the Lakeview residents' prior habitat stamped them as a naturally occurring affinity bonded group. Their new domicile seeks to synthesize every incoming resident into a neighbourly milieu of comparable affordable comfort, intellectual stimulation, social activity and special events. An interactive process of formal and informal care evolved over time. It involves a community activities director, a unique educational gerontologist–counsellor, and a representative group of the Residents' Association. In concert with the health care specialists of the community, they weave a web of trusting interpersonal connections between the new resident, old residents and staff.

Since its inception 17 years ago, the Lakeview community has become a stable place of entrances and departures of persons in their third and 'fourth age' of life (von Mering, 1992b). Altogether, the residents and staff epitomize a socially supportive, well-being oriented and also personally liberating environment to age and die in. As a community of elders, Lakeview is an example of the power of careful thought and open learning over the mere perception of the negative realities of ageing. It creates avenues for new growth and hope during advanced longevity. It is a community by cultural origin, choice and necessity that cares.

PART NINE
Integrated services

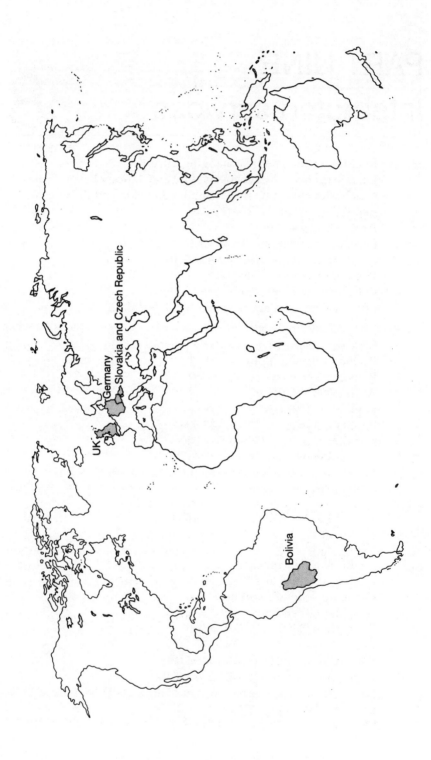

Integrating services in a changing Europe 28

A Czech and Slovakian perception

Jan Reban and Antony Bayer

The fragmented political and economic map of Europe which emerged after the Second World War has changed dramatically in recent years. The growth of the European Community and the re-emergence of democracy in central and eastern Europe gives hope for a new, more integrated Europe of nations sharing experiences and with common ideals, yet all dedicated to retaining their individual cultural inheritance. In place of the Cold War atmosphere of mutual suspicion and antagonism, there is a developing spirit of co-operation and respect. This provides both challenge and opportunity for developing innovative systems of health and social care, closer collaboration between professionals from many varied backgrounds and objective cross-national research in areas which previously may have been considered too politically sensitive.

Within this new Europe it is the elderly who represent the fastest growing political class, with both a relative and absolute increase in numbers of old people as well as an ageing of the elderly population itself. For those in northern and western Europe the demographic pressures are already being felt, whereas in southern and eastern Europe their effects are only just beginning to have a significant impact.

Thus by the year 2025, current projections suggest that nearly every country in Europe, with the exceptions of only Romania, Albania and Ireland, will have at least one in five of their population of pensionable age. The great majority, as now, will be living at home but with fewer younger family members available and prepared to be primarily responsible for any necessary day-to-day care or supervision.

Fortunately increased life expectancy is not inevitably associated with universal ill health, significant disability and constant need for medical and nursing care. Most old people are active, independent and self-reliant. Furthermore, relative health among the aged has improved considerably in the past 20 years, presumably because those factors, largely environmental, which increase life expectancy also tend to reduce morbidity. The elderly of the next century will have had the benefit of health education programmes when young and so stand to reap the benefits of not smoking, better diet, regular exercise and so on. Certainly the expectations and needs of the 80 year olds of the future may be very different from those of today. Nevertheless, despite these encouraging trends, the use of health and social services is considerable in old age and the growth in absolute numbers of elderly people seems likely to place them under increasing demand.

Attitudes towards the care of the old have long been determined by the health of the economy, the general standard of living and the overall state of morale within society. Neglect and maltreatment in previous years may be more easily understood within the context of past history. In the future there can be less justification for ignoring the special needs of older people or following a policy of merely banishing them to institutions when demands are considered too great. The growing affluence of many European countries and a more understanding and positive approach towards those members of society least able to help themselves should encourage the development of a readily accessible and integrated system of primarily community based medical and social care, freely available to all, regardless of age.

SERVICES FOR THE ELDERLY

Efficient health care delivery and provision of appropriate social services to older patients must be provided on an anticipatory as well as a demand led basis. The primary care team will play the central role in delivering this service, providing a readily accessible, comprehensive system of initial assessment, followed by coordinated, multidisciplinary care, support and education of patients and their families within the local community. It is importantly also the gatekeeper and key to more specialized services and by timely referral is often the major influence on ultimate outcome.

Access to the whole range of hospital based services should be freely available to all, regardless of chronological age, whenever they are needed. A specialist in geriatric medicine will be of particular value when illness develops and symptoms are atypical and in the presence of multiple pathology and polypharmacy. This is especially so when physical and mental illness is combined.

Alongside the health based services there should be a wide range of mainly community based social services, capable of adapting to the very different and often changing needs of elderly people and their carers.

Whilst the principle of keeping elderly people at home whenever practicable is central to good management, a minority will always require the special resources of institutional care. The emphasis must then be on demedicalizing and normalizing the environment, so that residents can have optimal social and psychological care as well as appropriate medical and nursing management.

The voluntary sector, newly established in post-Communist central and eastern Europe, can also play a vital role in care, complementing but independent from the statutory services, highlighting gaps in service provision and developing new approaches to solving unmet need. The lack of bureaucratic restraints allows them the flexibility to be innovative, initiating new developments and then pressurizing the authorities to take over responsibility if and when this becomes appropriate.

When planning delivery of services to the elderly, it is important to realize that a change in functional competence, for example withdrawal from usual social activities or a deterioration in self-care, does not always indicate a need for social rather than medical intervention. There may often be an underlying medical problem which may not be immediately apparent, but may well be readily treatable. Certainly, significant dependency is uncommonly a consequence of the ageing process itself. Curative care (for example, treating the breathlessness of heart failure, incontinence secondary to urinary infection, or forgetfulness due to depressive illness) may thus sometimes be more appropriate than the more immediately obvious solution of introducing prosthetic support services (home care workers, laundry services, supervised day care).

The introduction of social services, and certainly admission to institutional care, should therefore always be preceded by a comprehensive assessment of medical, social and psychological state. Services can then be carefully tailored to the needs of the individual, rather than the individual being made to fit the service. This will require an integrated system of care, with a close working relationship between health and social services, hospital and community, statutory and voluntary sectors.

Ideally all services for the elderly, both health and social care based, should be coordinated by a single authority with eligibility being assessed on an individual basis, generally by primary care doctors or case managers. When assessment and needs are more complex, clients should then be able to be referred on to specialist geriatric assessment teams who can ensure that intervention is optimized. Such a two-tier system helps to limit the costs of care planning which can otherwise be prohibitive. Funding must be flexible, so that money can be rapidly redistributed within the whole of the system according to changing needs and priorities.

NO PERFECT MODEL YET

The countries of Europe have in the past developed varied systems of care for the elderly, differing in form and emphasis. None would yet claim to have devised a model which is comprehensive, widely available and generally affordable. Many are still fighting a legacy of negative attitudes towards their older citizens, with few relevant community services and poor quality institutional care as often the only viable alternative to care by and within the family. Particular difficulties arise in those countries without nationalized health care systems, when financial fears may deter older people from seeking help until problems have become well entrenched. In eastern Europe, current economic changes are already especially disadvantaging the elderly and there must be concern that planned reforms of the health and social care systems will further compromise their position.

No country in Europe officially condones ageist health care policies, but segregation or prioritization on the basis of chronological age and to the detriment of the old is still widely practised. However, a growing number of studies are now proving that appropriately selected older patients can benefit from 'high technology' medicine and surgery as much as the young and long held prejudices are increasingly being challenged. The emergence over the last 30 years of the specialty of geriatric medicine has done much to highlight the benefits of active management of illness in old age and to introduce innovative approaches to care. In the UK, its activities and influence are now an established part of National Health Service provision for older patients, as well as a model for the development of geriatric medical services around the world.

Home visiting by doctors to old people also remains a feature of the British scene, with about two thirds of consultations with the very old taking place at home. Indeed, the new general practitioner contract now requires an offer of a home visit to be made at least annually to all patients aged 75 years or more for a medical and functional assessment.

In contrast to the general absence of home visits by doctors, home nursing is still carried out to varying degrees in many European countries. In Slovakia and the Czech Republic, specialist 'geriatric nurses' were long employed to provide a regular surveillance programme for all old people living in their catchment area, monitoring health problems, checking blood pressure and performing simple urine and blood tests, as well as assessing social conditions, functional independence and need for additional care or supervision. Whether they will survive current reforms remains to be seen.

The provision of a well-established system of high quality social care is an essential complement to good medical care. The availability of particular services, however, currently varies greatly between countries. For example, in Denmark 17% of those aged over 65 years receive home help, compared with only 7% in France and less than 1% in Italy. In Scandinavia, social care networks are particularly well developed with, for example, even rural postmen being used to check on old people and alert Social Services where needed. Despite the differences in availability of home and community based services across Europe, there is universal interest in non-institutional alternatives for provision of long term care. Some countries, including Germany, Sweden and the UK, give limited financial assistance to informal carers looking after elderly relatives at home and increasingly formal screening mechanisms are being used to control admission to institutional care.

While certain principles of service provision will be relevant to all countries, solutions to problems in one cannot automatically be expected to be equally successful in another. Nor must the transfer of experience be always in one direction. There are strengths and weaknesses in the system of care for the elderly in all the countries of Europe, including those previously under Communist rule, and all have much to learn from each other.

SHARING INFORMATION

Recent political changes across Europe have provided an unprecedented opportunity to develop and exchange ideas concerning the organization and practice of health and social care for the elderly. There is a general awareness of the urgent need for a coordinated response to the social, political and economic pressures of the growing numbers of elderly people in Europe. Moreover, the benefits of sharing information and experience are now widely accepted.

The European Exchange Centre for Gerontology (EECG) was therefore established in 1991 in Ceske Budejovice in southern Bohemia as a forum for discussion, research and training in the field of geriatric and gerontological care. The central geographical position, the well-established traditions of elderly care in Slovakia and the Czech Republic and the close links with other gerontological centres and organizations were decisive in its development.

The main objectives of the EECG in its first years are:

1. to establish a network of collaborating centres and experts from across Europe, to exchange information and to promote and stimulate gerontological research and cross-national studies. Special attention will be paid to the problems of cross-cultural assessment and the need for standardized measures;
2. to gather and store information concerning the problems of the elderly in Europe and successful examples of approaches to their care. This information will then be readily available to interested professionals, researchers and planners;

3. to organize short term courses on all aspects of care for the elderly and to encourage and arrange exchange visits between professionals;
4. to co-operate with government and non-governmental organizations concerned with the elderly, especially those seeking European integration and to facilitate and encourage collaborative developments;
5. to collect funds necessary for the implementation of these activities and with a view to providing financial support to future research and innovative developments in geriatric care.

The initial activities of the EECG have mainly centred on developing links with other European organizations concerned with the elderly and in the preparation of joint meetings and publications. The European Federation for the Welfare of the Elderly (EURAG) has been encouraged to open a new centre for central and eastern Europe, based with the EECG, and a successful EURAG conference has been held in Slovakia and the Czech Republic, with participants from over 20 European countries. The EECG has also helped HelpAge International to organize a workshop in Prague concerning the development of voluntary organizations for the elderly in eastern Europe and other similar initiatives are planned.

With the support of the WHO Healthy Ageing Programme, a collaborative project in the field of memory problems and early dementia has also been started, based initially in centres in Cardiff (Wales), C. Budejovice (Czech Republic) and Grenoble (France). The Community Memory Project, based on the experience gained over the last few years by a team at the University of Wales College of Medicine, involves the early identification, multidisciplinary assessment and management of elderly patients living at home with memory and related problems, especially early dementia. Such patients are largely dependent on relatives and friends and they require easy access to effective, flexible and preventively oriented, community based services specifically designed to address their special needs. Medical, psychological, nursing and social work services must be closely integrated, so that patients and carers are assured of comprehensive assessment and support throughout the course of the illness.

It is hoped that the development of the Community Memory Project may act as a model for interdisciplinary care, not only for those with memory problems but also for the development of integrated services for incontinence, immobility and other major problems of the old. Varied social, cultural, economic and environmental conditions will inevitably require alternative systems of care to be developed and evaluated, but each country should learn from its neighbours. Together they can build an efficient and quality service for their older citizens, closely integrated with other components of the national health and social system and ensuring continuity and equality of care and optimum use of all available resources.

Extending services of an elderly persons' home

29

Hogar Sagrado Corazon, Trinidad, Beni, Bolivia

Sister Pacifica McKenna with Ken Tout

The problems of ageing in a society disrupted by migration are now well known. For an elderly person with no pension rights, to lose the support of the extended family in a remote developing country region can mean a life sentence of extreme suffering or even an early death sentence. Mass migration is usually associated either with out-of-country movement, such as from the Caribbean to the USA or the UK, or else into one of the huge new 'megacities' like Mexico City or Bombay. In fact it can have a disastrous impact on individuals in smaller settlements.

Trinidad town, although the capital of the Bolivian Department (Province) of Beni, has much of the aspect of a 'frontier town', with a population of less than 50 000 and the possibility still of being totally cut off from the rest of the country at certain times. Until recently there was no all-weather road into Trinidad. The great Beni river could rise and flood the area, including the airport. Or the river could recede in drought times so that the normal boat communications could be closed down.

The vast region reaching to the Brazilian border is partially hostile open plains, with cattle ranching requiring extreme toughness in its employees, and partially jungle-style forests where itinerant rubber tappers work in difficult conditions for little profit. When a person becomes too old to tolerate such daily tasks the only hope of refuge is found in the tiny central town of Trinidad, at the Sacred Heart home. And it is likely that younger members of the family will have migrated far away, into the Andes Mountains around La Paz, or to some other country.

It was in the late 1970s that Sister Pacifica, already a veteran of 40 years service in Beni, heard of and approached the London organization Help the Aged, appealing for a small sum of cash to repair the leaking roof of the small Sagrado Corazon home. The appeal produced a visit from Dr Ken Tout who was studying the possibility of Help the Aged's involvement in Latin American age care programmes.

THE ONLY ELDERS' RESOURCE

At the time demands on the hard-pressed health services were so acute that it was decided not to admit to a hospital ward anyone over 50 years of age. Treatment might be given but then the patient must be accommodated elsewhere. The only public resource was the 26-bed home, housed in two long low pavilions, both needing some repair against the rigours of the tropical climate. In order to fit 26 beds into the space available it was necessary to push beds much more closely together than nurse–sister Pacifica would have wished. All types of terminal and chronic cases had to be catered for in the confined space. Communal activities were carried on upon the narrow verandah whose original purpose was as a rain barrier for the actual buildings.

A first planning meeting recognized that, with some ground area being vacant between the two buildings, an extra pavilion should be constructed as soon as possible. Given the economic realities and the service urgency the first plans were prepared using a foot rule and a penny exercise book! However, it was mutually agreed that any such extension should immediately provide for some kind of service to elderly of the local community who, although not resident, were perhaps in worse extremes of poverty, hunger and abandonment than the lucky if cramped residents.

Sister Pacifica, among her other abilities, was also a trained physiotherapist. In Trinidad, physiotherapy was not the somewhat leisurely or preferred option that it might sometimes be considered to be in more fortunate countries. An old person living alone in Beni had to be mobile enough to work, or at least to beg and visit charity points, in order to eat and survive. Physical rehabilitation was therefore a basic requirement of survival. So space was provided for residents and non-residents to undergo practical rehabilitation.

When meals had been served on the crowded verandah, cooking was carried out for the large resident family under heroic conditions in a tiny leaf-and-straw roofed hut. Now there would be an adequate kitchen which would offer the hope of providing meals also for indigent non-residents. The ample dining room could be adapted for useful activities. An instance both of the poverty of residents and their ingenious activities was the old man who manufactured mud pellets. Many local families supplemented their meagre diets with dishes of wild birds which were killed by the simplest possible means, that of throwing missiles at them.

But there was a method of manufacturing a mud pellet of such a dimension and shape that it could be propelled more accurately and thus help to improve a family's inadequate nutrition. The new pavilion would give space and opportunity for residents to take up more technical income generating activities such as shoe repairing or tailoring.

Sister Pacifica had at one time been the town midwife, as she had also been founder of a school and of a leprosy rehabilitation centre. Some of the babies she had brought into the world and some of the infants she had taught were now citizens who came to support the new venture as Help the Aged funds supplied the skeleton building. They formed an action group which followed the project's objectives of extending service into the general community. A parish priest at a distant locality persuaded the local military regiment (not notoriously committed to charitable enterprise at that time) to construct another feeding centre for elders alongside the church. Military officers organized a Field Day to raise much needed additional funds.

With the support of the enthusiastic local bishop, himself well beyond regulation retirement age, and the Catholic charity Caritas, a stable system of food provision was organized, both for feeding centres and for individual distribution. Within two years some eight varying activities for the elderly had sprung up, some in Trinidad town and others in rural villages. A local surgeon, Dr Eloy Avila, became head of the local group and was then instrumental in encouraging other Bolivian cities to take up the same age care ideas, to a point where a national association could be formed with Dr Avila as president.

Meanwhile, one of Sister Pacifica's colleagues, a young Spanish nun, had become a little impatient with the slow development of the one-by-one individual income generating activities. Having observed the Bolivian women's genius for the production of colourful woven products, such as shawls, ponchos, bags and carpets, she envisaged a more rapid and commercial application of the income generating project. Taking advantage of another international visit, with now some 16 varying activities to be seen locally, she proposed the donation of a weaving loom of commercial standard at which elderly women could, on a rota basis, take turns in weaving a little extra income, both for themselves and for the project in general. She had already established some very effective home made pottery kilns (the kilns, as well as the pottery being home made!).

For an almost insignificant sum of money, in international terms, a cottage industry style wooden weaving loom was procured and shipped to Trinidad. Inspired by their young leader, the local church youth group decided they could improve even further on the project. They took the loom to pieces to find out how it worked, successfully put it back together again and then constructed another ten similar looms from wood obtained by their own efforts from local forests. In a number of tiny huts and cottages the entire domestic life was now dominated by a large loom standing on the dirt floor, with an elderly woman weaving away at intricate patterns in brilliant networks of thread.

Interested in further publicity for the project, the nun heard of a national exhibition of traditional arts and crafts to be held in La Paz. Taking some of the products from the looms she went to La Paz and asked permission to display the goods. To her amazement the judges awarded the first prize in weaving to her elderly collaborators, even although they had not officially entered the competition!

A TIDE OF INITIATIVES

Other initiatives were equally attractive. One day centre, 'built' in a jungle village, was to be 'opened' by an international visitor. On arrival it proved to be a thatched roof supported on four stout poles, but no walls, doors or windows. It was already 'open' to the elements. Nevertheless, it was the possession of the elders of the village and, having a simple kitchen, it could be hired out by the elders to any other group wishing to use it at convenient times.

The result of this veritable tide of initiatives was that the Help the Aged headquarters in London agreed to include the Beni organization, now using the name Pro Vida, in the very sensitive Adopt-a-Gran programme. This system, by which donors in 'The North' support specific individuals of 'The South', requires extremely sensitive assessment of cases, judicious selection of benefits and careful monitoring of monetary input. Here, in a very remote region of the world at the headwaters of the Amazon, the entirely voluntary organization had proved itself capable of providing such a structure, thus introducing invaluable support for older persons in an area where an earlier visit had recorded elders as dying in extreme suffering because of lack of funds for simple medical treatment.

The increase in attention given to problems of the elderly soon made it apparent that physicians needed more knowledge of the peculiar physical and psychological conditions which very old persons might develop. Dr Walter Moreno had worked enthusiastically with Sister Pacifica but had no formal geriatric training. Neither was there access to such training nationally at the time. It was therefore necessary to arrange a placement for the doctor at a geriatric hospital in Brazil, the only one of its kind for literally thousands of miles in some directions. On return, in addition to tending patients with more insight as to geriatric conditions, the doctor immediately put his new knowledge to training others. Trinidad, almost the humblest of departmental capital 'cities' in Bolivia (Pando is the smallest department of all), had by now been selected by the other Pro Vida groups as the national centre for Pro Vida Bolivia for two years. The national secretariat (all volunteers) was to rotate to other departments on a two year basis. The Trinidad group therefore had a significant contribution to make nationally, as well as later entertaining visitors from other Latin American countries who were interested in rural age care strategies.

As a crowning piece to this structure of innovation, HelpAge International secured funding so that an appropriate multifunctional day centre, with outpatient facilities and more activities rooms, could be erected on the Hogar Sagrado Corazon's old cocoa plantation. This has already proved such a magnificent central resource that Sister Pacifica did not mourn the destruction of her cocoa plantation, which never made a profit. With the former pavilions now fully used for residential purposes and a new matron in charge, Sister Pacifica, now in her 80s, has time to spare to make regular visits to elderly persons in the surrounding community and exercise her many skills, her latest innovation being a new ophthalmic programme for elders.

It was in 1964 that Sister Pacifica's collaborators had begun building the first dormitory pavilion. By 1979 the roof was leaking. In 1985 the British Ambassador opened the new additional pavilion. Then in five years the tiny project had become town-wide, region-wide, nation-wide and was even inspiring visitors from beyond the frontiers.

An important feature of the entire Beni programme is the extent to which volunteers can initiate and maintain an age care programme up to a certain level of demand. In this case a regular group of some 35 volunteers, supported by more casual volunteers as necessary, has been able to cater for the most urgent needs of a constituency of between 300 and 400 persons aged from about 55 upwards, with rarely more than two nominally fulltime staff and two nuns coordinating the various enterprises at at least 16 centres. A considerable proportion of volunteers, including the veteran Sister Pacifica, have been of what might be termed 'mature age'.

Another lesson emerging from the assessed range of needs is that older persons continuing to live in a relatively stable and undisturbed rural society are not to be considered as exempt from the impact of family breakdown. Endemic rural poverty exacerbated by societal breakdown can mean extreme suffering for certain distressed individuals.

On a more practical note, a warning alarm was sounded through the weaving scheme already mentioned. The unplanned provision of a number of looms meant that, when other areas contemplated replicating this excellent project, they had to be dissuaded, because the Beni looms had saturated the available national market for such products. The pitfalls on the road to successful income generation are many and often not immediately evident.

Sister Pacifica herself emphasizes the less material aspects of the story: the faith which sent the original request letter off 'into the blue'; the disciplined commitment which arises from a personal creed of service to 'my neighbour'; and the frequently expressed desire of older people for spiritual support and consolation, especially in moments of bereavement, which is an aspect often overlooked in the more rigid requirements of international grant aid procedures. In this area of concern one of the most frequently expressed needs of elders is for the assurance of a decent funeral with attendant rites, and this is something Sister Pacifica can now promise more happily than when she had to 'knock up' burial boxes with her own hands from odd pieces of lumber. And use the boxes for successive burials!

A multifacet centre   **30**

Report on the first two years' development of Queens Park Court, Billericay, Essex, UK

Jai Tout

The Basildon Social Services Area of Essex County Council includes the towns of Basildon, Billericay and Wickford. As in the rest of the UK the numbers of elderly persons are increasing, from 20 253 in 1981 to 27 332 in 1991 and an estimated 30 494 in 1996. In the town of Billericay the increase over the period will be 38.1% compared with 33.6% for the area as a whole.

A 1982 survey revealed a waiting list of 33 persons for Elderly Persons' Residential Part III accommodation, plus 370 persons already using intensive home help services (who could be described as potential elderly persons' homes (EPHs) users), as against an admission capacity to existing EPHs of only 32.5 per year in that period. A later calculation showed 52.5% of persons requiring such accommodation to be women on their own, as compared with 17% of men on their own.

An unusual feature of the Basildon population is that growth was developed through the establishment, post-World War II, of a 'new town' to draw off workers from distressed areas of London. These workers were actively encouraged to bring their parents with them to maintain family links. However, over a period, some of the workers migrated further afield in search of better careers, leaving their elders often isolated in relatively unfamiliar surroundings.

THREE AUTHORITIES COMBINE

That need directed thinking to what in the UK was, at the time, an unusual collaboration. Three authorities, which generally worked independently of each other, agreed to combine in the establishment of a new style multipurpose centre in a developing community area of Billericay called Queens Park. The three authorities were Essex County Council (responsible for Social Services), Basildon District Council (responsible for housing), and Basildon and Thurrock Health Authority (responsible for health care).

A capital cost of £3.5 million was accepted and a firm contract agreed, under which the authorities allocated the responsibilities which each would undertake, such as Basildon District Council taking on routine property maintenance, whilst Essex County Council provided lighting, heating and communications. A proportional breakdown of common revenue costs was also enshrined in the contract.

The site available was 3.244 acres in extent. On this was constructed a complex including 30 Category 1 sheltered housing units (for the more active); 30 Category 2 units (for less active); four 'bungalows', each with ten beds of Part III provision, these being linked by an enclosed glazed street; a resource centre including social work offices and medical consulting room; restaurant and kitchen; activities centre large enough for dances; shop and bar; quiet room; craft room; launderette and plant rooms; staff room; offices; health and beauty salon; stores and central WCs.

The Part III bungalows, named consistently with the title of Queens Park Court after houses of the royal family, were 'Kent' affording accommodation for persons mentally alert but physically frail; 'Gloucester' for the mentally alert but moderately able; 'Windsor' for the very frail both mentally and physically; and 'York' for planned respite support.

As this complex was opened and developed from 1989 onwards, it was able to offer a multifocus support service from the reassuring presence of a 'warden' for Category 1 units to 24-hour close support in the 'Windsor' bungalow. The sheltered housing warden had duties extended to that of a liaison officer to facilitate the use by the Category 1 and 2 residents of all the communal facilities.

Non-resident day care elders of the local community had access also to the communal services whilst intergenerational relationships were encouraged by opening restaurant and coffee bar to relatives and friends. Residents could eat in their own units or use the communal meals service which was not restricted to the tight time schedules often imposed in residential settings.

Health Service district nursing staff gave an average of 22 hours weekly attention to residents in their own units. The resource centre provided further services in dentistry, ophthalmology, physiotherapy, chiropody, occupational therapy, welfare advice and group meetings. A formal day centre service was set up five days a week with ten daily places for local non-residents who had been assessed as having needs which could be met by a certain number of daily attendances each week. The location of a community team of social workers on the complex meant that not only was there a convenient outreach to non-residents in this area which was still being built, but the team was able to provide a substantial home help service into Category 1 and 2 units.

MULTIDISCIPLINARY STAFF

Staffing necessarily had to be multidisciplinary. The liaison officers were being asked to undertake roles beyond that usual in sheltered schemes. Care staff in the bungalows were expected to implement new regimes of independence and freedom of choice to persons who would hitherto have been considered to be recipients of imposed care disciplines. 'Support' was the preferred practice term, rather than 'care'. Risk was accepted as necessary at times in the interest of a person's continuing independence, whilst that independence and self-care were prominent preventive measures against confusion.

Staff members being recruited were expected to bring four essential qualities, irrespective of paper qualifications: experience, management skills (for senior staff), interpersonal skills and empathy with the elderly. An intensive and rigorous five day induction course enabled new staff to understand the philosophy and developing practice methods within the centre. The initial induction was followed by appropriate in house training as well as access to external courses.

The key worker role was introduced so that residents might have the confidence of relating to a well-known supporter. However, in order to provide continuity of such confidence, the key worker system was extended to provide two care workers who, on a rota basis, would share a special relationship with an elderly person, thus reducing the off-duty gaps when a single key worker would have been absent.

Referral of elderly persons from the community for possible residence at the centre can be initiated by the prospective service user, the family, the general practitioner, a specialist consultant, the district nurse, the local hospital and others. The response to referral is a home visit and assessment by a specially trained social worker, using a common instrument for interview and recording. A multi-agency panel considers the case and a possible 'package' of services.

A trial residence period can introduce the elder to EPH conditions – another centre, The Woodards, having facilities for this. Family discussion and visits to Queens Park Court are integral steps. Should the person be admitted to the complex as a resident, there is a review at the end of six weeks to assess the suitability of the provision.

To deal with the referral process a multidisciplinary panel was set up to consider appropriate service users. The panel included a district nursing sister, a community psychiatric nurse, a home help organizer, a social worker, a housing officer and an occupational therapist.

From handover of the centre by the builders, the immediate management of all the complex's services was exercised by a manager who was a qualified social worker, appointed by the Social Service Department in liaison with the other authorities. The District Council appointed the liaison officers for Category 1 and 2 accommodation. The overall responsibility for multidisciplinary collaboration rested with the Principal Officer, Elderly Services, of the County Council Social Services Area Office.

From the date of inauguration of services, performance reviews were instituted on both an internal and external basis. These reviews covered both the evolving centre procedures and actual standards of care achieved. The elderly residents were also involved in the process of review, contributing useful criticisms as well as welcome plaudits. Indeed, residents' opinions were most seriously considered, so that an eventual review result of 90% highly satisfied residents was no great surprise. And the 10% expressing some grounds for dissatisfaction were concerned about relatively minor aspects such as lack of storage space, inadequate extractor fans and the need for adaptations to showers.

RESIDENTS' INDEPENDENCE

Independence and choice were enhanced by such measures as the requirement for staff to knock on bedroom doors before entering; the need for any visitor – irrespective of hierarchy – to obtain residents' permission to enter units or bungalows; the ability to eat, bath and perform natural functions in private, as and when desired; the freedom to dress to one's own taste; and not be bound to a 'rota' system of getting up and early evening retirement. This was in accordance with the practice of freedom of choice implemented throughout the local Social Service department area.

Residents happily joined in real opportunities for planning the more leisured aspects of central life, especially the organizing of special events and open days. Initiatives were constantly displayed whether in the Easter Bonnet parades or individually, as when one tenant living in the sheltered housing area undertook a five mile sponsored walk without leaving the complex, completing 30 circuits of the corridors to raise £150 for special causes.

Reality orientation was a particular aspect of staff discipline, including such mundane actions as constantly reminding confused residents as to time, place and persons; allowing time for hesitant responses; and composing clear simple answers and instructions. There was high take-up of craft and other activities. A University of the Third Age activity was introduced, offering educational opportunities to persons of retirement age.

The manager appointed was an accredited practice teacher qualified to line manage and teach students for the CQSW (Certificate of Qualification for Social Workers). From 1990 such students have taken up placement at Queens Park Court, coming from both official services and the private sector.

Local community volunteers furthered the policy of integration of the complex into local life. The volunteers, reacting to the royal title of the complex and district, and observing the atmosphere of fun and enjoyment expressed by residents in their activities, soon gave themselves the name of 'The Court Jesters'. Their services were both serious and entertaining, ranging from shopping trips to gardening and writing letters for residents, as well as helping in the major events.

Another stratum of volunteers involved younger people. School pupils made a very much appreciated and exhibited video recording of an open day. Children entered a competition to design a logo for the Court Jesters. Senior pupils carried out an excellent evaluation of the volunteer system.

Spiritual needs are most important to many elderly people. Local clergy and lay volunteers were available to bring spiritual comfort where needed. A monthly inhouse religious service involved all local churches. Volunteers maintained a 'get you to church' service. The local church Cub pack (junior Scouts) entertained residents.

Such a massive material project, with its practice innovations and interpersonal complexities, could not move into full operation without some problems, delays and doubts. Senior managers from the key agencies met on a monthly basis to receive reports from the site managers, evaluate progress, resolve interagency difficulties and generally advise and direct on developments, the Social Services personnel again holding the central coordinating brief.

Very soon overseas visitors found their way to Queens Park Court as a possible model for replication. Such visitors were fascinated by one aspect of the programme. During much of the planning and development periods the County Council was in the hands of one political party whilst the District Council was of another political persuasion with normally conflicting policies. The Health Authority, deriving from the national ministry, was a different type of infrastructure and had differing procedures, to say nothing of the traditional misunder-standings which could occur among varying professional specialities. Yet, amid all these diversities, the Queens Park Centre collaboration achieved common cause with no major disruption due to varying initial opinions.

Early contact was made with the local media and information was openly dispensed, with several press conferences and access for special articles to be written. This resulted in the still-evolving local com-munity being well aware of the nature and purpose of Queens Park Court, whilst practical support was drawn from the wider catchment area. A member of the royal family, HRH the Princess Royal (Princess Anne), was eventually able to perform an official opening ceremony with the centre in full running order. The Princess was interested to know that the names of their units had been chosen by the residents themselves.

PROBLEMS AND SENSITIVITIES

One of the most serious problems encountered was that the theoretical staff ratios invoked in the early planning and budget stages proved to be insufficient once all the services and procedures of the complex had been decided and calculated. In the interim dependency levels had changed and would continue to fluctuate, demanding variations in provision. The requirement in some units for 24-hour, seven days a week (and, less obviously, 365 days a year) cover strained the limits of the theoretical measures. Night lifting in emergencies was one such factor, with its geographical and human resource implications in a large complex where more than one emergency might occur at the same 'out-of-hours' time.

Staff stress was another factor which had to be forecast and possibly prevented by adequate training and supervision, such time consuming requirements being the alternative to high rates of staff absence through sickness due to stress. The very high dependency conditions in some units required correspondingly high concentration of effort by staff, whilst the insistence on independence as far as humanly possible, together with a planned acceptance of certain risks, did not always enable the speediest discharge of staff duties.

There was also a considerable early tension between the habits of wandering on the part of confused residents and the requirements of freedom of choice in personal programmes. Staff trained to more rigid regimes found it initially difficult to cope with unscheduled, randomly staggered rising, eating, dressing, bathing and bedding permutations. At a later date they discovered that this uncertainty of timetables had the effect of long term easing of normal interpersonal tensions, both staff-to-resident and staff-to-staff. For the efficient operation of the centre, the emotional needs of staff generally are a most important consideration.

A subtle but important aspect of centre life was the fact that, far from isolating the areas where permanent 24-hour care might be necessary, the interdependency of centre facilities gave able Category 1 residents a 'window' – in more ways than one – on the happy experience with dignity, choice and privacy enjoyed by those who were more frail or confused. The sensitive preservation of independence in high dependency areas and the emphasis on empathy to the exclusion of enforced discipline proved to have high morale value for more able residents.

A further factor of potential conflict was in the very willingness and eagerness of local volunteers to become involved in this outstanding programme within their own community. The volunteers' need to serve was, in some cases, adversely encroaching on the residents' ownership of the locale and sense of ability to decide on minute details of life. At the same time a volunteer, often serving at some cost to his or her own convenience, required a task equal to the commitment. Otherwise the fountain of goodwill could easily dry up.

Over the development period it was eventually agreed that the efficient running of the Part III and communal services segments of the complex would require a considerable, well trained Social Services staff. This would comprise the manager, a senior assistant manager, then 97.5 hours weekly of assistant manager time, 78 hours senior care assistant, 199.5 hours night care assistant (with an assistant manager sleeping in), 572 hours care assistant (day), 291 hours domestic assistant, 95 hours cook, 37 hours clerical and 39 hours driver/general handyman.

The Category 1 and 2 sections are served by two liaison officers, whilst the whole complex enjoys the services, as already indicated, of district nurses, other Health Authority staff and input as appropriate from the community team of Social Services.

An innovative project needs a clear philosophy. This has been described as 'a safe supporting environment where residents can live life to the full in ... freedom, friendship and fun – where each person is an individual retaining dignity, independence, freedom of choice and control over their own lives'.

In the important consideration of retaining a stable, competent staff group, the philosophy is 'to build a close knit team of carers and the cared for; living and working together; maintaining relationships and always offering one another the hand of friendship, tolerance and respect ... to offer the staff opportunity to recognize their own skills and talents through a management policy of training, supervision and support'.

Wedding the incompatibles

31

Using counselling services to mediate between formal and informal care

Kai Leichsenring and Birgit Pruckner (Germany)
(Linguistic editing: Suzanna Stephens)

Counselling services for frail elderly people and their family caregivers are considered to have become more and more important in many European countries. In Germany, there are at least five reasons for this trend:

1. the priority given to home based care for the elderly;
2. the growing pluralism of care providers and the lack of coordination between them;
3. an underdeveloped service culture, especially in rural areas;
4. a new interplay between formal and informal help and care;
5. increasing demands for self-determination and control by both users and relatives.

Information and counselling have played a minor role as long as services remained relatively undifferentiated, easy to survey and part of a well-known local environment (e.g. the local residential home or community nurse) and formal help and care services were called in at a very late stage when informal care networks either could no longer cope or had collapsed and professionals were called upon to make the 'necessary decisions'.

COMPLEXITY OF SERVICES

However, the landscape of providers of services (voluntary organizations, commercial providers and care initiatives) has become increasingly varied and complex – and so have the legal entitlements and modalities regulating the use of services. A further factor involves the increase in home and day care services: the interplay between the formal and informal sectors, formerly a sequential one, has come to be not only an important but also a constant issue.

Professional services have never been able to take over the bulk of informal care provided by the family and only recently have they explicitly supplemented and supported it, thereby considering the informal carer as an active co-producer. In this process, services are seen less and less as emergency interventions, rather becoming issues of choice and individual 'packaging' where users and their informal carers demand a say. In this process, the social competences of the elderly person and his/her carers gain an impact. On the basis of a comprehensive knowledge of their rights and options, as well as of the practical constraints, they seek not only to achieve a tailor made care arrangement but also to retain control over this arrangement. So far, service providers have failed to meet this need for information on the part of clients and informal carers.

There are several factors which have influenced the set of motives and normative values of informal carers: higher mobility, overall individualization and the generalized participation of women in the labour market. These factors all affect their ability to take on responsibilities by caring for their partners or family members. The specific type of 'care' which family caregivers will be able and willing to provide in the future will be advocacy, mediating activities, negotiating and supervising care arrangements. This development and the attitudes that are linked to it have so far not been adequately considered by the formal care sector.

On the one hand, however, an open minded approach to services has taken shape while on the other, there still exists a widespread fear and reluctance to use professional help and care. The attitudes towards service consumption range between family members conceiving themselves as advocates of their dependents by arranging appropriate services (which was discussed above) and the traditional caring spouse who only accepts support for special, mostly medical tasks. Especially in rural areas and among elderly spouses, it is often seen as a personal failure and disgrace to resort to public services.

Given this background, several counselling centres have been set up as model projects in different German regions. We have chosen three examples from Bielefeld, Augsburg and Marburg in order to illustrate their ways of mediating between formal and informal care. They differ considerably with respect to their conceptual framework, aims, focus of activity and organizational structures – as will be shown in the following. While the counselling service in Bielefeld still exists, the model project at Augsburg has not been continued and the Marburg centre has been transformed into a local division office for elderly policies.

THE BIELEFELD PSYCHOGERIATRIC COUNSELLING CENTRE

The growing number of mentally ill or elderly people suffering from dementia makes particularly high demands on informal care networks, being the main reason for their breakdown. This is usually followed by the institutionalization of the elderly person – a disastrous chain reaction if we consider the vital impact of a familiar environment on the health and well-being of this particular group. The counselling centre in Bielefeld was set up with the explicit aim of enabling people suffering from dementia to remain in their own homes by providing advice and support to their informal carers. These are addressed in a double role. Firstly, elderly clients are not in most cases able to consult the agency themselves; rather, they depend on a mediating person – usually the caring relative – who acts on their behalf and attends to their special needs. Secondly, family caregivers themselves have to cope with immense physical demands as well as emotional stress and strain. It is not unusual for them to become isolated or trapped in a destructive caring relationship. Care professionals are usually both overtaxed and helpless when faced with the burn-out of informal carers; they rather tend to ignore them. In contrast, counsellors particularly focus on these needs.

In a sense, this model experiment represents among the examples considered a more traditional and limited approach to counselling. Although the network of services is part of its mediating activities, it is primarily concerned with individual clients and their acute problems. This may partly be due to its relatively weak position *vis-à-vis* service providers. The centre was set up in 1990 by Evangelisches Johanneswerk, a church affiliated non-profit organization. Thus it is neither independent nor authorized to coordinate care provision for the elderly. It was added to a quite well-developed infrastructure of Social Services – including home care services – and could build on the pre-existing loose networks of care professionals in the district. Most of them welcomed the new advisory service because they expected it to relieve them of 'caring for the carers' – a task which they were badly prepared for and rather reluctant to take on themselves, as mentioned before. The bureau was accommodated inside a residential home – a fact that proved to be advantageous, as many carers turned to the home for help when they could no longer cope on their own.

The counsellors – a social worker and a social trainer – promoted the project by initiating public debates on the issues of 'ageing' and 'care giving', as well as by networking services and institutions concerned with the elderly. Many activities – as for instance, organizing working groups on topics of shared interest – intended to advance both cooperation between a variety of providers and professionals and a needs oriented service culture. Though the centre's ability to coordinate existing care facilities depends on the goodwill of service providers, it has succeeded in establishing a continuing dialogue both on quality criteria for services and on care needs of elderly people suffering from dementia among local care professionals.

In the daily routine of the centre, however, the focus is on individual consultations, i.e. providing information and counselling that enable family carers to deal better with their situation. This may also include an unbureaucratic mediation and 'packaging' of services, advice on financial matters and questions of housing, or long term psychological support. Increasingly, too, care professionals seek advice on basic knowledge regarding the psychiatric diseases of elderly persons. In addition to this consultancy service, which is actively marketed by different channels, the counsellors offer training courses to professional, voluntary and informal helpers as well as supervision to self-help groups of carers.

However, most carers do not consult the agency unless faced with an acute crisis that requires quick intervention. Under such conditions, it is rarely possible to work out the most acceptable care arrangement with all persons involved; but relief, rather than empowerment, can be gained by opening up limited choices for carers, e.g. helping them to escape isolation, or to master feelings of resentment or guilt towards the dependent person.

THE AUGSBURG PSYCHOGERIATRIC COUNSELLING CENTRE

A decisive factor for setting up a counselling centre in the Frankonian city of Augsburg had been the local 'development plan for the elderly'. Because of the dramatic increase in people in need of help and care, the issue of care could no longer be dealt with as a matter of private family tasks. The counselling centre was run as a model project, financed by different German foundations, with the aim of making the problems of dependants and their carers an issue of public interest.

One of the main characteristics of the counselling centre in Augsburg was that its multiple aims did not only include fostering information and mediating different services for the elderly. Above all, the counsellors tried to build a solid network of services, clients and policy makers so as to introduce new approaches in the planning process as well as in the provision and utilization of services. The living conditions and the social problems of dependent people were introduced to different political committees and planning bodies (e.g. for building, cultural activities or health provision). Several projects in these areas were realized: for instance, consultancy for the adaptation of apartments or houses to the needs of gerontopsychiatric clients, special education towards an activation and rehabilitation of persons suffering from dementia, information exchange among the elderly or 'holidays instead of psychiatry' for informal carers.

Apart from the provision of decent information, a process needed to be launched in order to create public awareness of all matters linked to care and psychogeriatrics in the community. Nevertheless, this process had to be organized in a sensitive way, by trying to influence the prevailing attitudes of professional service providers as well as those of family carers. The providers had to become aware of the necessity of designing new services oriented towards consumers' interests, by offering more flexibility and by acknowledging the important role of family carers in the caring process. With respect to the users, it was very important to support them in articulating their needs as well as to alleviate fears, reservations and feelings of guilt that were often linked to the use of services.

The two counsellors who had previously been working in other areas of help for the elderly had already started to develop the project by an analysis of the existing service structures. The comparison between existing structures and needs articulated by clients showed an obvious mismatch between supply and demand – be it quantitatively or in terms of quality. Relevant factors were the shortage of day centres, inflexible time schedules for service providers, lack of training or supervision for staff and lack of understanding of the informal carers' own need for support.

The analysis resulted in establishing a constant dialogue with the providers of services, based on daily contacts with the counselling service centre's clients. New services, such as day centres, were developed in cooperation with the municipal administration, private non-profit organizations and potential clients to overcome identified shortcomings. Other activities, such as courses for carers, seminars for the professional staff in community care or working groups on qualification and training, served as a starting point for confidential relationships and fruitful co-operation.

In spite of the counselling centre's having worked in a highly innovative and efficient way, the model project was urged to stop its activities after three years of service: its budget could no longer be secured. Now both the municipal administration and the private non-profit organizations will be forced to increase their direct responsibility for stabilizing existing networks and for establishing user-friendly information points within their own organizational structures. Nevertheless, a precondition for the centre's success had been its independent position: usually administrative structures – as well as service providers – tend to pursue their own interest, having no opportunity to mediate between each other. So far, they have not thought in terms of holistic approaches. The future will show whether they may manage to effectively take over the function of an independent counselling centre, one free to create a solid network for dependent people and their carers.

THE MARBURG CARE ADVISORY BUREAU

In contrast to the previous examples, the care advisory bureau of Marburg operated in a rural area where the myth of a well-functioning and self-sustaining system of family care for elderly people was still upheld. That this was no longer a reality – if it had ever been – was drastically pointed out by a preceding study on the changing social relations of elderly people in rural areas. With this study, two counsellors had laid the analytical foundations for this consultancy service, run as a model project for two years and financed by the Robert Bosch Foundation.

Based on interviews with elderly persons and their family caregivers, important sociological knowledge was gained on living and care arrange-ments of elderly persons. The most striking result was that the moral norms and expectations of the (older) population clearly contrasted with the sociostructural changes of the past decades. There still prevailed a culture of caring obligations and privacy, but there is also a rather negative image of services, particularly among elderly people, which provoked strong reluctance to use public services or to share care tasks with professional helpers. The majority of service providers reflected these barriers by carrying on paternalistic traditions rooted in a professional care system offering help to 'helpless' people – thereby reinforcing the stigmatizing effect of service consumption.

Given this background, the counselling service aimed at bridging the gap between the private worlds of caring and professional services. Potential users had to become more aware and to see things in an evaluative light.

- Caring is not a problem to be solved within the private realm of the family but rather calls for a fair public share of responsibility.
- It is therefore a legitimate strategy to use services.
- Providers have to reorganize service delivery in such a way as to be sensitive to the needs and fears of clients.
- Local policy makers need to recognize that the issue of care for the elderly presents a major challenge for community policies.

As personal consultations would have already presupposed an active search for public support on the part of the clients, counsellors at the centre depended on extensive public relations in order to reach their target group, i.e. elderly and their carers. They used local newspapers, started educational and media campaigns and experimented with imaginative forms of public relations, all of which particularly respected the personal anonymity of clients and raised awareness for the plight of family carers.

At the end of the model experiment, an expert meeting was convened to discuss future perspectives on ageing and care for the elderly in rural areas. Impressed by the great international interest and by the outcomes of the conference, the district government authorized the counsellors to elaborate a comprehensive concept for care policies in the district, as well as to set up a local division office for policies on ageing.

However, the further financing of the advisory bureau could not be secured. Due to the lack of adequate services, e.g. day or respite care, and to the unwillingness of providers to co-operate, it had reached its structural limits, too. Particularly when trying to coordinate existing institutions, services and care professionals, the counsellors had met with considerable resistance: the voluntary organizations were more preoccupied with **not** interfering with one another. It was only a logical consequence to focus further work on influencing their attitudes in the first place. Thus, the experiences of the counselling service helped to formulate the aims of the local division office – to initiate a collective process of reorientation among service providers, to overcome an uncoordinated service development and to make care for the elderly an issue of public policy.

CONCLUSIONS

The spread of counselling services for dependent people and their carers must be seen in relation to the development of specific service cultures in different welfare states. In the Nordic countries of Europe, the use of social services is already a well-known part of daily living but in continental welfare states (e.g. Germany and Austria), the overall scarcity of such services, as well as their proximity to social assistance schemes, still creates opposition to talk of developing a similar service culture. Especially in those countries where care has been mainly conceived as a private task of the family and where services have been provided in a patchy and rather unplanned manner, counselling services – or other agencies dealing with information and coordination of existing services – are of growing importance. Still, the question is whether counselling services will be able to establish a network prepared to serve clients' needs in practice or if they only play a cover-up role in between political divisions and the legitimate interests of strong voluntary non-profit organizations.

Certainly, counselling services are the potential 'pioneers' of a new service culture. Thus, they have also to experience the limits of their intentions within an environment characterized by an overall scarcity of resources. Apart from that, new actors in any given system are not at all welcomed at first sight, especially if they are trying to change existing structures and routines. Depending on the goodwill of local policy makers and service providers to co-operate with them, counsellors generally have to face a difficult and time consuming process. With respect to their potential clients, they have to deal with prejudices existing within informal care relationships *vis-à-vis* the use of external help, or with the disappointment of carers with respect to the existing services. As a result, the existing structures and prejudices – both on the side of the services and on the side of the informal carers – must regrettably be recognized as a vicious circle with which counselling services have to deal on a continual basis.

The examples of Augsburg, Bielefeld and Marburg have illustrated the first steps to overcoming this vicious circle by means of a sensitive moderation of public debates, political decision making and individual advocacy. By developing a network between actors and institutions – which so far have not been co-operating – counselling services may become mediators between authorities, providers and users of services. In the beginning, this mediation may only be akin to crisis management. Still, in the long run, the integration of dependent people and their carers will be indispensable in the planning process of care arrangements supported by special agencies. If this does not happen, then 'pluralism', 'choice' and 'help for self-help' will be no more than catchwords in the realm of public debates on community care.

PART TEN
Within the Mind

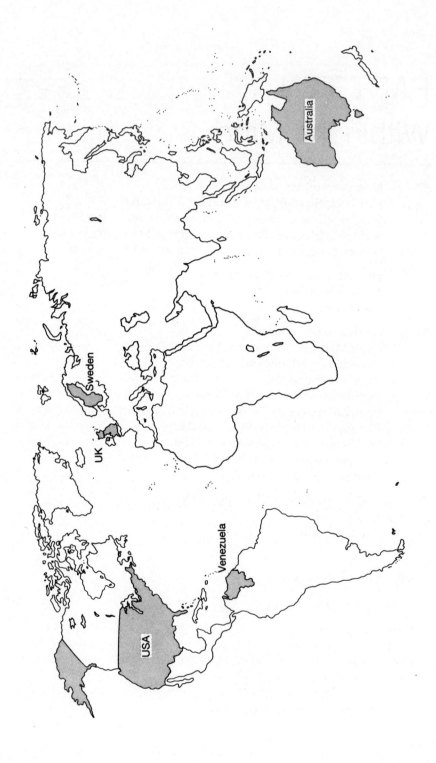

New perceptions of dementia

32

Some selected advances in concepts and social practice (Sweden, USA, Scotland, Australia)

Ken Tout

At a recent Alzheimer's disease conference in the USA I was commenting that, in certain developing countries visited, there appeared to be no clear comprehension on the part of some physicians and nurses – to say nothing of family carers – of the various causes and probable courses of what is often termed confusion or 'dementia' or mental deterioration with ageing. I was astonished when my North American counterpart replied, 'You could say that of quite a few physicians and nurses here in the States'.

The psychogeriatric discipline is a comparatively young field of study and experiment but one which has tremendous implications for misunderstood elderly persons who might enjoy a much fuller and better life than they do, as might also their carers.

A SWEDISH DEFINITION

The Swedish psychogeriatrician, C.G. Gottfries, comments:

> Historically, dementia indicated a progressive disorder. This is no longer so. Some dementias may remain stable for years, or progress to a final stage in which the patient may live for a shorter or longer time. A fluctuating course is also possible. Furthermore, it is unacceptable to define dementia as an irreversible clinical condition. There are forms that are reversible.
>
> (Gottfries, 1991)

He also clarifies 'secondary dementias' which 'can be divided into dementias due to intoxications, infections or immune disturbances, metabolic and endocrine disturbances, nutritional disturbances, expansive processes, disturbances of cerebrospinal fluid flow, trauma and stress'. He claims that 'dementia can be a manifestation of hysterical or conversion reactions'. If this appears to be a wideranging definition it at least illustrates the vast field of possible error open to the unwary, uninformed, unqualified family carer or volunteer helper.

It might therefore be thought inappropriate to publicize systems of 'self-evaluation' such as the 'Nuremberg Self-Evaluation List'. However, under expert guidance these are now seen as an integral part of the process of diagnosis and monitoring. It is especially useful for routine screening and early diagnosis of incipient problems which can be examined and treated, rather than left to cause later anxiety to carers and further problems to practitioners.

The Nuremberg questionnaire does not consist of 'relating to a momentary state, but asking for a comparison with the past' and is based on the assumption that 'the persons concerned are the first to perceive any changes in their everyday life'. Indicators are of the nature of 'recently I have tended to put off uncompleted work; recently I have frequently mixed up names, telephone numbers or the date; recently I have tended to have more difficulties in planning a trip or other activities' (Oswald and Gunzelmann, 1992).

Obviously, as already implied, such instruments need to be used under close practitioner control as the simple phenomenon of confusing a telephone number might easily cause an untrained, unsupervised subject to assume the imminent onset of Alzheimer's disease, ignoring the fact that people of all ages confuse such numbers. An answer to a single question is only valid as a part of a very much larger sum and as part of a historical comparison process.

AUSTRALIAN HOME CARE

Later in this review there is a reference to training of carers in Australia, but first it is instructive to look at the official provisions made for dementia care in the home in Australia. From 1985 legislation has enabled the setting up of the Home and Community Care Programme. Within a broader remit special consideration is given to certain highly specific groups including the ethnic aged, older Aborigines and those with dementia. The aim is, through more comprehensive domiciliary support, to enable members of these groups to remain with more independence in their own homes and avoid inappropriate admission to institutions.

The programme is carer oriented and its five categories and sets of services have been defined as:

1. helping the carer manage: the Domiciliary Nursing Care Benefit, information and advisory services and counselling, including carer groups, education and training, and case management;
2. assisting the carer with practical tasks: home help, personal care, domiciliary nursing, transport, home maintenance and modifications;
3. providing relief from caring: respite services in the home or in day centres, complementing the provision of respite in nursing homes and hostels;
4. getting more from the system: assessment, information and advisory services, advocacy services and user rights strategies;
5. services provided to the dependant: include all the direct care and support services listed above (McCallum and Howe, 1992).

In addition to the central programme there was also a Community Options component which was commonwealth funded 'to foster innovative approaches to service delivery, especially for individuals with complex care needs' and 'to enable the "packaging" of services' to give the most flexible response to individual requirements.

SWEDISH DEMENTIA APARTMENTS

A Swedish initiative provides special group dwellings for dementia patients, which have all the appearances of normal apartments within a building in the community but with an outside lock to ensure security. Preferably it is a ground floor location. There is 'either a "cluster" of apartments (usually six to eight) or a small group of dwellings with shared premises. Each resident has an apartment or a room (with a toilet and shower) of his or her own and use of a common kitchen and living room' (Johansson, 1990).

Furnishings can be brought from the residents' former homes. All fixtures are designed to merge into the atmosphere of a normal family home but consideration is given to the need for dementia sufferers to be able to orientate themselves easily.

> Staffing density varies from 0.5 care personnel per patient to 1.2, with an average of 0.9 according to severity of dementia. Each resident has a designated 'contact person' among the staff who serves as a 'stand-in' family member. The contact person has primary responsibility for the personal care and the psychosocial well-being of the resident.
>
> *(Johansson, 1990)*

This type of accommodation is being urgently evaluated for further replication because Sweden envisages the need for about 30 000 such places by the year 2000. The problems arising so far include the perennial query of residential establishments as to what to do when the condition of the resident (or the cohort) deteriorates to a level of dependency beyond that for which the existing programme is currently planned and budgeted. Would it be possible to retain a highly demented, bed ridden person within this family sized community of persons of limited competence? And what about the resident whose psychiatric condition exhibits complicated symptoms beyond the 'normal' dementia for which the programme has capability?

NEW TECHNOLOGY

Perhaps it is not too soon in the evolution of psychogeriatrics to take a brief look at what the future of technological invention may offer for dementia sufferers. The Robotics Institute in Pittsburgh is one of the forward-looking centres which offers to translate space age systems into domestic tools in the near future, to ease the burdens of trained nurses and family carers alike.

It is good that the director of the laboratory there can say:

> The informal caregiver (family, friends) plays a significant part in caring for and maintaining the older person at home . . . their need for assistive technology is as great as or greater than the formal caregivers' . . . As numerous informal caregivers become frail themselves the needs for alternative methods of care provision, such as assistive technology, will intensify.
>
> (*Engelhardt, 1989*)

Among the objectives of invention and research are those of:

> surveillance and monitoring: this area is a chronic problem for caregivers . . . who are plagued by wandering behaviour and falls. Our research specified a system that could utilize space technologies such as satellites to track wanderers and artificial intelligence techniques within the environment to locate and if necessary communicate with the wanderer.
>
> (*ibid*)

Already there is the capability of installing a 'mind jogger' which can be programmed to emit messages in the caregiver's voice and can transmit other signals to help orientate and rouse the person where the more formal stimulus of a persistent carer is absent. Engelhardt's concept of a 'smart home', a living space totally geared and equipped to the dementia sufferer's requirement, would help by 'optimizing the use of residual abilities, compensating for lost capabilities . . . enhancing, augmenting, or extending typical human capabilities' (but see comments in Chapter 44).

The ability of non-formal carers actually to cope and to care is fundamental to the welfare of persons suffering from dementia for the foreseeable future. Research suggests that caregivers who were caring for care receivers with a high degree of memory and behaviour problems were more stressed, more burdened and less able to cope than those concerned with lower degrees of memory and behaviour problems in dementia. It also suggested that caregivers did not receive enough social support, that as many as 30% might be having serious problems of care management and that nine out of ten caregivers were looking after the elderly person fundamentally because there was no alternative available (Kwan, 1991).

SCOTTISH MISCONCEPTIONS

A number of research projects into aspects of dementia have been carried out in Scotland recently and one of them concentrated on the average carer's attitudes. A problem existed because many carers do not make themselves known, carrying on their family service without linking into external networks, so that it is difficult for researchers to produce a precise profile of the 'average carer'.

The particular research project found a large number of carers convinced that dementia was a kind of social death; 66% of the carers felt that 'It is as if he/she is already dead', whilst 55% agreed that 'Death might come as a blessing to him/her', referring, of course, to the care receiver. One carer stated explicitly, 'You say to yourself, "Oh my God, if he would just go to his bed some night and I woke up in the morning and discovered he was away" – then I would say "What a relief!"' (Sweeting, 1991).

Giving more data along the same lines, the researchers concluded: 'having established the confidence of the carer it is usually possible to talk about these issues with them . . . several carers were relieved to hear that they were not the only one to have had "bad thoughts" about the event of the dementia sufferer's death'.

In a sense the untrained carer can be like the soldier on the field of battle who, at the moment of crisis, senses extreme fear and thinks himself a coward because he is unaware that almost everybody else is equally scared. In the face of much very honest reaction to surveys like that cited, the need for urgent training of carers is evident, especially in cases of dementia. Indeed, as Sweeting and others point out, conscious and constant efforts have to be exerted to find and identify the carers in the first place.

SYDNEY TRAINING INNOVATION

An Australian report is significant because it touches upon both the efficacy of training care givers for cases of dementia and the financial logic of supporting informal care, rather than allowing a deterioration which will eventually require much more expensive services, as calculated by the investigators.

The training course in question took place in Sydney. In the first of three groups, a ten day intensive course at a teaching hospital was undertaken by pairs consisting of a dementia patient and his/her carer. The course covered medical, legal, financial, welfare, dietary and nursing themes, as well as group psychotherapy experience. The carer also received tuition in reality orientation, behaviour modification, therapeutic activities and reminiscence therapy. The problem of 'carer burn-out' was considered and there was active support for setting up or enlarging a family/neighbour network to further support the carer.

As a control for this intensively trained group, two other groups were trained, one being a patient-only course and the other a delayed patient and carer programme. The experimental project as such covered 100 pairs.

The significant evaluation has taken place 39 months after the training. This allowed both for an extended period of carer–patient relationship and a sufficient period for the purposes of accurate comparative costings. Twenty two of the patients were dead by this time but their deaths constituted an important segment of the data. Of the patients still alive and living at home, 55% were from the first early pair course, 38% from the delayed pair course and only 13% from the patient-only course.

The researchers summed up their extensive findings in these words.

- The comprehensive training programme for carers reported here was associated with an increased likelihood of patients remaining at home and, as a corollary, a lower rate of admission to institutions.
- Carer training appears to be associated with a lower mortality rate and this may be an indirect effect resulting from the reduced rate of institutional admission.
- Carer training can be cost effective, as these results have been achieved with significant financial savings to the community, as well as with significant reductions to carers' psychological distress – and therefore ability to continue caring (Brodaty and Peters, 1992).

Hidden wealth within dementia

33

Testing the combination of reminiscence therapy with counselling skills as a new approach

Marie Mills (UK)

Dementia is a disease that is comprised of a series of 'cannots'. The patient has poor short term memory – can**not** remember the immediate past; the patient can**not** manage his or her personal hygiene; the patient can**not** manage to remain in the family home without support.

The impact of dementia on the individual is, therefore, a series of accumulative losses such as diminished cognitive functioning leading to loss of memory and individuality. As the illness progresses, most sufferers will need long term support, possibly funded through community care budgets and/or residential care.

The implication may be that they lose their home and, certainly, their former way of life. The process of dementia can be seen as a state of powerlessness and lack of control over one's destiny. It is, in many ways, the loss of a life.

Much is known of the negative effects of this illness but is this the only way of viewing dementia?

SOME MISUNDERSTANDING

Irreversible dementia is not merely a disease caused by biological changes in the brain. It is an illness that has psychological and social processes which 'give good reason to believe that social and psychological factors influence symptom formation and the course of dementia' (Hanley and Hodge, 1984). Thus this is a multifactorial and multifaceted illness which affects a substantial and increasing proportion of the elderly population. The literature indicates that the numbers of elderly sufferers of dementia are increasing.

Much of the literature on dementia tends to focus on the behavioural aspects of this illness and/or changes in brain function which would explain these alterations in behaviour. Very little is written of the psychological impact of this disease which causes this behaviour, but the proven case for demonstrating the cause of dementia as organic does not rule out any psychological processes that may precipitate or generate such biological changes.

Much of the reminiscence work with demented elderly people has focused on an area in which the older person, albeit with dementia, is an acknowledged victor. These older people have lived longer than their researchers. They have experienced past events that are only possible for the researchers to understand via secondary methods. Enabling older demented people to recall their past through group reminiscence therapy is one way of seeing and understanding the person behind the dementia but there is also an increasing trend to study the approach used by therapists in these sessions. This approach recommends the use of Rogerian techniques such as unconditional positive regard, empathy and attentive listening.

Some recent research, undertaken by this author has indicated that individual reminiscence therapy combined with counselling skills allows the demented person to recall more fully significant past life events. Not only did this group of people recall the factual content of these memories but also the emotions associated with these experiences (Mills, 1991). The use of counselling skills enabled them to share their feelings with another person in a more equal relationship. This approach allowed the investigator, who was trained in some aspects of counselling techniques, to understand the meaning and significance of the informants' recalled past and to feel a greater understanding of them as individual people.

The study investigated the ability of five elderly people with severe dementia, who lived in a long stay psychogeriatric setting, to recall/review their past lives. The only criterion was that these people should be able to speak and would enjoy the experience of talking to another person. The interviews took place once a week with a total of 21 recorded and transcribed interviews. These varied in length from approximately 20 minutes to one hour.

SOME CASE STUDIES

All informants identified major themes during the interviews. The most common theme was that of loss/change and the denial of loss/change.

One informant could not understand why he no longer saw his friend of many years. He referred to this frequently during our interviews.

SL. 'He sort of went out of my life ....Disappeared out of sight. We fell apart then.'

He denied strongly that his friend had died.

SL. 'Oh no, he didn't get ill, nothing like that! I forget exactly what happened.'

His experiences during the war were meaningful for him, especially seeing/losing many of his comrades, killed at Dunkirk.

Another informant, throughout the interviews, indicated that he did not feel a 'whole person'. He felt that he had rarely managed to meet his mother's high standards. When I said his mother must have been proud of him, he replied,

CF. 'I suppose so, yes she must have been. She didn't show it much.'

He lost his father at a young age.

CF. 'It was a hard life especially losing the father.'

The increasing loss of bodily control due to old age concerned him.

CF. 'You're never confident in yourself. Always appear to be ashamed of yourself. You see wetting the bed, etc. It ... ah ... appears to be terrible.'

The staff on the ward had told me that this informant would sometimes wander the ward looking for his school cap, which he felt he had lost. He had said during the interviews that this article of school uniform was regularly checked by his mother.

CF. 'A blooming blue and gold cap which if you lost cost five bob, I suppose, I don't know. It was a precious thing really. Mother used to check that blessed hat. If it had a mark on it, you got nagged about it.'

Yet another informant spoke about loss in her life. She spoke of her first husband with great affection. He was very dear to her.

AL. 'Oh yes! Oh yes, a dear! Oh dear, it makes me feel dreadful when I think of him you know!'

She nursed her parents until the end.

AL. 'Yes that's right. Oh they were a lovely couple! And of course then they died, you see.'

One informant always denied loss in his life. On one occasion during my visit to the ward he was wandering along the corridor. I asked him if

I could speak to him. He said that he was going out.

AR. 'Well, I'm just on my way up to the village.'

He agreed that I could walk with him and by the time we reached the day room he had forgotten his desire to physically revisit the place of his childhood.

He still saw his father as working in his brick factory.

MM. 'So your father was the manager of the brickworks in ———.'

AR. 'Yes. He still is. Up at the brickworks.'

When I asked him if he had been fond of his father, he replied,

AR. 'Oh yes! I still like him .... Still works up at the brick factory.'

This denial of the death of a parent has been the subject of a Dutch thesis on the phenomenon of parent fixation in some elderly demented persons. Miesen argues that parent fixation is a key to the experiential world of the demented elderly in which more or less permanent feelings of unsafety trigger attachment behaviours (Miesen, 1990).

IMPORTANT INTERACTIONS

All informants had stories to tell that involved one or more of these categories. Our personal identities are created through interaction and our actions are shaped through our social interaction with others. It is possible to argue that all interaction, including interaction with ourselves, occurs in a 'place' and that this is an event or happening. These interactions or relationships with others, places or events are important to us all.

This description of these relationships helps us to understand and accept the 'world of the other'. It meets the goal of the interpreter in his or her efforts to make the invisible visible to others.

This description of the experiences of the informants enabled the investigator to understand and share these experiences. Their emotions reached out and touched the listener. When Mr L. described his feelings on seeing the vessel that was to remove him from the beach at Dunkirk, one, too, felt the relief at being rescued from a place of terror.

SL. 'I'll always remember it. She poked her nose right through the burning dock and brought us home.'

Mr F. also enabled others to share his world. When he described his childhood, it was possible to feel great sorrow for this small boy who tried so hard to please his mother.

CF. 'I did my best ...... Generally! .... Sometimes!'

Mr R., in describing his childhood, created pictures of a way of life that sounded loving, safe and warm. One could imagine what it was like to live in a closeknit community with such parents who sounded wonderful.

AR. 'Well I've got, I've got a ...a magazine here and a book. He'll [his father] read this today, tonight. He'll lie in his chair there, and read away with the gas light just above him.'

These stories suggest that reminiscence work with some elderly confused people plus the use of interviewer counselling skills can be beneficial to some elderly who are demented. This therapy allowed the investigator to enter the dim dark world of the demented person. It may allow others to discover the locked door of some memories that have meaning for the older person.

The importance of memories is manifold. Memories enable us to perceive ourselves as individuals with our own individual experiences. The recalling of past memories for the informants enabled them to remember, albeit briefly, the people they once were.

Mr L. recalled with pride his part played during the war. He was a lance corporal in the British Expeditionary Force. He recalled his army number; it was 196743.

Mr F. recalled the various jobs that he had had. He was asked about his teaching career.

MM. 'You became a school teacher didn't you?'

CF. 'Oh my dear girl! I've done ... er ... become all sorts of things! Been an engineer. I've been ... oh ... chemist ..... chemical analyst and all sorts of things!'

Mr F. sounded rather like a school teacher as he spoke.

Mrs L. recalled her interest in amateur dramatics.

AL. 'I loved acting, yes. I loved it in every way.'

Mr R. remembered his life as a reporter. He said it was a good job and paid well.

AR. 'I was on the ———— Courant and the ———— Times.'

He enjoyed his work especially on the Courant, as the chief reporter was a friend from his village.

AR. 'He was with us ... chatting away all the time.'

It can allow the demented person to recall memories that need to be evaluated for the life review process and share the 'hurt' of obsessive past episodes.

SHARING PAIN

One of the greatest gifts we can give to another human being is the willingness to share their emotional pain. Mr L. was hurt because he no longer saw his friend Fred Drummond. He sounded lost and bewildered as he said,

SL. 'He sort of went out of my life.'

Mr F. felt very 'unworthy' most of the time. He did not feel that he had pleased his mother when he was young. He had a very poor self image. He did not think he was a good person, yet his wife had said that he had been a good husband and father. He had provided well for her.

MM. 'Do you think you have had a happy life?'

Mr F. thought about this for a while. He sounded regretful as he spoke.

CF. 'Weighing it up and looking back, I shouldn't think so, no.'

On another occasion he spoke about religious beliefs.

MM. 'Do you think you are a good person?'

There was a long pause. Mr F. whispered his reply,

CF. 'No!'

Recalled and described memories also allowed individual informants to become a 'storyteller'/teacher to the young. Mr R., possibly because of his reporting career, was a natural storyteller. The senior charge nurse had spoken of informants' interests, but these were never successful topics for interviews. Most informants would answer questions concerning these supposed interests but with evident lack of interest.

Mr R. was no exception. He wanted to tell his stories and they developed as the interview progressed. He spoke on one occasion of the strong beer made in his part of the world. Mr R. often had a drink after work with his fellow reporters.

MM. 'It's quite strong isn't it?'

AR. 'Yes! When you've had a few pints you didn't notice!'

He would travel back to his village either by bus or on the train. Often the call of nature became overwhelming!

MM. 'So you had to stop on the way home and spend a penny?'

Mr R. chuckled.

AR. 'Oh you'd tell the bus driver you wanted to go out of the win...winder and he'd make you get off the bus!'

SHARING LAUGHTER

All the informants were often intentionally funny. There was a great deal of laughter during the interviews. They seemed to enjoy this very much and it is possible to suggest that this approach, in its entirety, could allow the generation of more equal relationships that do not solely depend on the protective concern elicited by this type of illness.

It is possible that some of the strong emotions expressed by the elderly people during these interviews could have been overwhelming for someone without some knowledge of counselling strategies. It is a natural defence to 'block' or deny strong feelings in other people if the recipient feels unable, or inadequate, to cope with them. This can be a standard practice in the nursing milieu due to lack of training in counselling techniques and the pressure of the work.

This research indicates the beneficial use of counselling skills in psychogeriatric settings, especially amongst nursing staff. The possession of these skills would enhance the quality of care for confused elderly people. Counselling skills would enable the nurse/carer and demented person to converse in a more normal socially interactive manner.

The nurse/carer belongs to a group of 'interpersonal professionals' who spend most of their working life in face to face communication with others. The ability to communicate well with others is a crucial component of this work. As some individual interpersonal professionals are better social interactors than others, so too will the nurse/carer have better communication skills than older people with dementia.

Many of us who care for older confused elderly people perform certain personal care tasks that require private space and time. It is certainly possible to suggest that the use of appropriate counselling skills during these periods would lead to more effective communication. Thus the use of counselling techniques and counselling/reminiscence therapy could be incorporated into task specific interactions as a readily available, cost effective and enjoyable resource.

None of us may ever fully understand what it is like to have a dementing illness but we may gain some comprehension of the subjective world of the sufferer by trying to see the person behind the disease. This approach makes it possible for all caring professionals to gain an understanding and a new perspective on their patients. It merely requires some knowledge of the person's past and some basic coun- selling skills. It enables those of us who care for demented elderly people to actually talk to them and to discover a hidden wealth of rich feelings.

Recently I visited a psychogeriatric day hospital to assess a resident for additional community support. Whilst I was waiting for this lady to finish her therapy session I spoke to some of the other clients in the day room. Mrs B. told me of her past life and it was quickly established that, for her, the most significant and meaningful part of her life was when she was married and lived in London. She told me her husband was a wonderful man and that she missed him still.

Another lady described her childhood and her life in a small village in the country. They both told me that life was better for them then than it is today. These people are severely confused but their memories and feelings were valid. This small social interaction lasted perhaps ten minutes but I still recall our conversation with pleasure. The pleasure for them may have been momentary but it existed. Perhaps we should focus more on the moment with this client group and look to improving their quality of life and relationships.

This concept was highlighted during my research. One informant was thanked on completion of an interview. He asked why he was being thanked. I told him that our talk had been a pleasure and that he had looked happy whilst he was speaking to me about past events. This severely demented elderly man replied,

'And I tell you what! I felt happy when I was telling you about them.'

Note: This chapter is adapted from the article 'Dementia, Reminiscence and Counselling Skills: A New Approach', first published in *Generations Review (Journal of the British Society of Gerontology)* March 1992, and used here by kind permission of the Editors.

The impact of ageing amid sociocultural change in Venezuela

Luise Margolies

Old age, according to a recent article in the Venezuelan newspapers, is the only requisite for entering Purgatory. The aged population of Venezuela constitutes one of the smallest and least understood components of the Venezuelan population. Ignored and virtually invisible, the aged have barely captured the attention of researchers. Only two monographs have been written on this subject in the past 15 years, one by a sociologist (Aponte Bolivar, 1978) and the other by a geriatric physician (Mazzei Berti, 1988). Given the paltry state of knowledge, it is impossible to delineate the major characteristics of the Venezuelan aged. Nevertheless, I would like to discuss some of the critical changes that are currently affecting the ageing process for growing numbers of Venezuelans. As this group becomes more numerous, it will be impossible to ignore the demographic trends and their implications.

We are all aware of the worldwide tendency for the greying of national populations. According to UN estimates, the number of persons over 60 will increase by 57% compared with an increase of 38% for the total population. Even more impressive are the forecasts for the oldest old; those over 80 will burgeon by 70% as we move into the 21st century. In Venezuela, a developing petroleum-rich country in the midst of an economic recovery, such trends are already evident. The over-60s presently constitute 5.6% of the national population and are the fastest growing demographic cohort. Venezuelan society is still a young one, but the aged component will increase continuously, leading to the general ageing of the whole population.

The aged are a varied body. They are divided by differences in ethnic group, colour, rural/urban background, class and religion, national origin and occupational/educational levels. A diversity of ageing experience exists that does not necessarily crosscut the cultural boundaries of these various groups. But they have all been subjected to certain modern phenomena that have succeeded in transforming the entire ageing process. During the past few decades a few developmental factors have had such a sustained impact that successive generations of the ageing will have to deal with unprecedented ways of growing old.

AGEING IN THE CONTEXT OF A RURAL SOCIETY

The 1920s were a decisive decade for Venezuela because they marked the abrupt collapse of the traditional agrarian economy, to be replaced by one based on petroleum production. For nearly a century, the Venezuelan economy had depended on the rise and fall of its principal agro-export commodity, coffee. The nascent petroleum industry would engender a revolution in the countryside that within a 30 year span would transform Venezuela into a modern, urban nation.

Industrial capitalism provoked an enormous mobilization of the rural population toward the cities and permitted substantial investments in the public sphere. These developments produced immediate effects in the demographic profile. In the 1920s, Venezuela had a rural based population of only 2 411 952. Infectious and endemic diseases were rampant and life expectancy hovered around 30. The over-65 population was less than 1% (Mazzei Berti, 1988). Repeated public health campaigns led to declining mortality rates and a gradual increase in the natural growth rate. By 1949, when the *Patronato Nacional de Ancianos y Inválidos* was created, the population had doubled and the elderly sector, although still minuscule, now represented 2.3% of the total (Mazzei Berti, 1988).

In a reconstruction of elders' perceptions of ageing in a rural society, it is clear that growing old occurred entirely within a family and community context. The roles of the elderly could not be divorced from those of the rest of the family which functioned as an economic production group. Just as each stage in the family's developmental cycle signalled the assumption of new roles and statuses, ageing marked the final dimension of this ongoing process. Family members moved in and out of differing roles in accordance with their age and each step in the maturation cycle was accomplished smoothly. When ageing occurs under such conditions, as Fortes pointed out, 'Old age is ... marked by declining physical and mental powers but very often counter balanced by high generational status' (Fortes, 1984).

The rural family was an extended family group composed of several patrilineally related nuclear families residing in neighbouring households. Fathers, sons and brothers functioned as a co-operating labour pool and this kinship nexus was further reinforced by bonds of *compadrazgo* (fictive kinship). Extended family members knew that they could depend upon each other not only for economic tasks but for other forms of assistance as well.

Interpersonal relations within the family were governed by the rule of filial piety. From an early age, the children were instilled with the basic values of the rural family – to honour their parents, to honour their relatives, to honour their elders, and to honour their village. All relationships were put in terms of 'respect' and it was untenable for any household member to challenge the authority of the family head. The father was the owner of all economic resources and was the uncontested patriarch. In the hierarchy of authority, the wife had control over domestic matters, elder children wielded control over younger ones, males over females. The husband had the final say and thus, all lines of power were strictly drawn, leading always to the top.

To have as many children as God disposed was the guiding principle of the rural family – a large family with many sons was seen as insurance against the debility of old age. Children living in close proximity to their elders provided the ultimate security in the face of farming uncertainties and eventual infirmities. On a community level, familial norms of respect were further reinforced by an appreciation for the empirical knowledge accumulated by the elderly over a lifetime of hard work.

THE TRANSITION TO AN URBAN SOCIETY

Within a few short generations, the traditional institutions that moulded and insured the continuity of a rural way of life were irrevocably challenged by an urban order. Venezuela, apart from sustaining the highest urban growth rate in Latin America, has also attained one of the highest levels of urbanization in the continent.

The frantic pace of urban growth in Venezuela owes its momentum to three factors:

1. the dramatic increase in the natural growth rate over a 50 year period, from 10.5% in 1910 to 38.4% in 1960, as a result of rising birth rates (31.8% to 45%) and sharply falling mortality rates (21.3% to 7.5%);
2. the internal movement of the Venezuelan population in a pattern of rural–urban migration. The post-Depression years were characterized by the widespread exodus from the countryside as Venezuelans headed for the nation's capital, industrial centres and the petroleum states. In 1936, more than 70% of the population lived on the land but

by 1960, this same percentage was now concentrated in the urban areas;

3. the massive influx of European immigrants after World War II, which continued unabated for 20 years and was succeeded by a large influx from neighbouring Colombia, not only resulted in another doubling of the Venezuelan population between 1950 and 1970, but was directed primarily toward the urban areas.

Consistent with the rush to the cities are new values toward the land that undermine traditional extended family structures. For the generation that grew up in rural Venezuela, one's perceptions of an orderly world were conditioned by a commitment to family farming and the efficacy of empirically tested solutions. For the generation that came to maturity in the transitional period of rapid urbanization, the years spent in the countryside served as a gestation period for the erosion of obsolescent norms. The old pattern of large extended families living and working in close proximity was replaced by one in which children, one by one, departed for the city, leaving the elderly conjugal pair 'childless' once again.

The strict rules of propriety that ordered family relationships were only possible when socialization occurred within the confines of a family unit that stayed together in the same place. The 'loss of respect' that constitutes only one aspect of present intergenerational relations is merely one aspect of the conflicts produced by rapid sociocultural change. The elderly conjugal pair must now confront the demise of the traditional labour pool engendered by their children's migration. The reluctant departure of the elderly in their children's footsteps constitutes the extinction of the last residue of family organization that characterized the traditional agricultural enterprise.

THE AGED IN AN URBAN SOCIETY

Although there is still a good deal of disagreement regarding the 'pros' and 'cons' of modernization with respect to ageing, there's no doubt that the rapid development of Venezuela has had a negative impact on the position of the elderly in the national society. Paradoxically, the biological limits of ageing have been significantly stretched; not only has the Venezuelan life expectancy jumped from 54.20 to over 70 during the period of rapid development, but the growing numbers of elderly have access to more and better gerontological care than ever before. Yet both the concept of 'old' and attitudes toward the aged have dramatically changed – for the worse. One now grows old under the stigma of negative stereotypes in which ageing is a 'condition,' a 'problem,' even a disease.

Why has there been such a drastic revaluation of the ageing process? The primary reason seems to rest with the attenuation of the traditional roles of the contemporary elderly population. Before modernization, the aged performed their customary duties to the best of their abilities and received compensation in the form of intergenerational collaboration and care. Elders exerted control over productive resources, served in an advisory position for junior family members and participated, however nominally, in the unit's economic activities.

Today such roles are superfluous. The elderly are isolated from the economic mainstream of an urban industrial society that clamours for more and more technocrats in new and ever expanding esoteric fields of expertise. Laws and informal rules sanction this economic isolation; not only is the mandatory retirement age low, having been set when life expectancy was significantly lower (55 for women and 60 for men), but the workplace consistently discriminates against those over 35.

Social segregation is also rampant. Today, intergenerational conflicts are based on differing life experiences and ignorance of the maturation stages by the young characterize the ageing process. This situation is exacerbated by the physical dispersion of the former extended family due to rural–urban migration.

The Venezuelan situation is not unique. Ken Tout notes that everywhere under the influence of urbanization and internal migration, community values and respect for the aged pale in the new emphasis on putting the individual first. 'Whereas the extended family system is beneficial to the older person in rural areas,' he notes, 'the normal spatial family unit in the city becomes nuclear in capacity, while the old are seen as objects to be cared for by official services rather than being the prime concern of the family' (Tout, 1989).

Because of this socio-economic marginalization and the fact that the contemporary elderly are ill equipped to deal with the realities of an urban industrial society, attitudes toward the elderly border on the infamous. The stereotypic visions of the aged are uniformly pejorative and seem to be based on heresay and ignorance. All generations over 60 are indiscriminately clumped together as one amorphous unit and characterized in the most disdainful terms as weak, passive, helpless, sick, sorrowful, lonely, resigned and so on. The aged are treated as a dependent, non-productive burden on the rest of society and have even been considered to be 'disposable'. Visual images of the elderly in the media inevitably depict a sorrowful individual with a physical impediment, seated in a wheelchair, with insufficient dignity to be dressed. A horrendously wrinkled being, leaning on his/her hand with a look of utter resignation, completes the picture of the institutionalized, 'garbage dumps' for the nearly dead.

Such stereotypes commit a grave injustice by spreading false and simplistic notions of the ageing process. Not only do they lose sight of the enormous heterogeneity among the older population, but they lead to even more discrimination and social isolation in daily life.

Unfortunately, stereotypes are difficult to reverse and obfuscate actual realities. Today's elderly grew up in the 1920s and 1930s and were unprepared for the rapid urbanization and economic development of the country. This undermined their traditional economic and social roles. They also had the bad luck to grow old in unforeseen times, when a long recession, galloping inflation and a devalued currency eroded lifetime retirement plans. Nevertheless, recent analyses have indicated that contrary to popular opinion, nearly a third of the over-65 population is gainfully employed and living independently.

The elderly population has increased rapidly over the past decade, not only because of the healthful ageing of the entire population, but also because of the greying of numbers of Europeans that immigrated as youngsters in the 1950s and 1960s. Demographic estimations indicate that the over-75 group will grow more rapidly than any other, quadrupling by the year 2020, and the over-60s will burgeon to more than 3 million, constituting approximately 10% of the total population. Undoubtedly, this greying population will call for new permutations of social action and their demographic strength will make it difficult to dismiss them through derogatory remarks.

NEW APPROACHES TOWARD THE ELDERLY

Institutional care for the elderly in Venezuela has generally been based on the notion of a dependent group in need of custodial care. The early *casa hogares* (nursing homes) instituted by the *Patronato Nacional de Ancianos y Inválidos* in the 1960s were replaced by gerontological units that were meant to provide integral medical attention as well as residential facilities for the frail elderly. Today this national network of 27 units constitutes the central programme of the *Instituto Nacional de Geriatría y Gerontología* (INAGER). Approximately 50 000 elderly persons receive some form of service from INAGER, whose other programmes include ambulatory units and a pension programme for those persons not protected by the social security system.

Unfortunately, the nursing home model, one which has been emulated by both religious and private organizations as well, reinforces the pattern of segregating the elderly. Recent attempts to 'open up' the system of services (under the rubric of 'open attention') have been frustrated by bureaucratic delays, frequent turnover in personnel and drastic cuts in public spending necessitated by the debt crisis of the mid-1980s.

Venezuela is presently in a phase of economic recovery and privatization of services and industries. Clearly, the old welfare system will be unable to meet the needs of the greying population and there is a call for a complete restructuring. The institutionalization model is now being complemented by more dynamic programmes meant to improve the quality of life by addressing specific issues such as health, housing, recreation, etc. Under the motto 'give a hand to an elder', these programmes are a first step in addressing policies for the living rather than providing deposits for the dying.

Paradoxically, at a time when the demand for resources outstrips their availability, the Venezuelan population has a real possibility of facing ageing both 'resourcefully' and 'productively'. Elsewhere, I have dealt with the types of innovative programmes that will be required to renew the functional roles of the elderly within a family and community setting (Margolies, 1990); these include both grassroots movements and self-help projects that are cost efficient, easy to implement and based on the active collaboration of the elderly. The present greying population is well prepared to deal with the coming issues of the 21st century; they will be healthier, more active and more involved (Harootyan, 1991) than their predecessors. The growing empowerment of this group and its willingness to take collective action may provide the impetus for the nation to re-order its priorities, its policies and philosophy to promote positive ageing in the years ahead.

I would like to thank Dr Jesus Enrique Mazzei, president of the *Sociedad Venezolana de Geriatría y Gerontología* and former director of INAGER from 1969–74, as well as Lic. Felicia Saturno Hartt, former director of planification at INAGER, for their advice and suggestions regarding ageing issues in contemporary Venezuela.

The 'purgatory' piece appeared in an article entitled 'Mientras más años más desamparo' in *El Nacional*, September 10, 1984.

'Rage, rage against the dying of the light' 35

Caring in times of grief, loss and the moment of ultimate reality

Linda Machin

> Old age should burn and rave at close of day;
> Rage, rage against the dying of the light
>
> *(Dylan Thomas)*

The poignancy of this poetry encapsulates thoughts, feelings and responses with an economy of words and yet a richness of meaning that holds together some key themes within this chapter:

- the realities of loss as they escalate and accumulate in later years;
- the fiercely strong emotions which accompany loss;
- the pain of attempting a reconciliation between the (personally) acceptable and the unacceptable.

This is a reality which is often hidden behind the sanitized units of care which have marginalized, on society's behalf, the world of those no longer contributing visibly to the economic wealth of the community. To be an older person and to be experiencing loss is a double reason, in late 20th century Western society, to have one's concerns pushed to the margin. Whatever the pain and psychological struggle for those within this situation, the vigorous youth- and work-orientated world does not want to be reminded of its own vulnerability or ultimate destiny. It is safer to whistle in the sunshine and drown out the 'rage against the dying of the light'. For some older people, therefore, counselling can be one opportunity to find a creative chance to 'rage against the dying of the light' and restore dignity to life's experience at its ending, without the need to gentle to oblivion those struggles which themselves are manifestations of dynamic life.

What is the reality of the dying light and what is the rage that meets it?

INDIVIDUAL EXPERIENCE OF LOSS AND RESPONSES TO IT

What is it that inhibits the progress towards a satisfactory sense of fulfilment and maturity and obscures the visible recognition of these qualities for observers of the ageing process? That long life experience does not of itself produce a satisfactory self-view or world view is amply evidenced in situations of mental ill health and in some aspects of social malfunctioning in older people. Reactions may include:

- I can't cope (inadequate internal resources);
- I will be left alone (fear of abandonment predominates);
- I don't deserve support (poor self-image);
- What I know of the past leads me to be pessimistic about my present situation (inadequate support in the past);
- I may get even less attention for my grief if I stop being depressed (to be part of a support system there has to be a 'problem');
- My duty to my loved one demands that I keep my sadness alive (grief is bound to be chronic).

A lifetime of inadequately met need will produce some of the negative experiences within old age. Cumulative experience which has built on disabling messages, often given in childhood and reinforced by subsequent events, will have left an individual with the reverse filtering process to that of rose-coloured spectacles; life will be seen with a negative distortion which is likely to result in self-fulfilling prophecy of failure and disappointment. Where this has been the predominant pattern of experience grief reactions are likely to be chronic. A history of inadequate psychological and social resources will result in an overwhelming sense of being trapped in pain.

Within society there is an ambivalence towards old age which describes the ageing experience as one which might contain the best of all integrity or the worst of all disintegration. However, society is often passive in promoting the conditions which foster the former. The policy of care often remains located in meeting physiological needs and makes no progress in the less visible areas of psychological and spiritual need.

CHANGING AND LOSING: A FEATURE OF EXPERIENCE IN OLD AGE

It is possible to describe the origins of loss in two different dimensions; one through the sequential pattern of change (the life course) and the second through the less predictable and potentially more traumatic circumstances of:

- broken relationships;
- physical/mental illness/disability;
- economic disadvantage;
- unfulfilled aspirations (Machin, 1990).

What might this mean for an older person? In some ways there is a fusion of these dimensions as the trauma of an earlier age is incorporated into the pattern of change. Change is likely to bring profound rather than gradual shifts in life circumstance. Losses may be multiple and the physical and emotional resourcefulness to meet these may be potentially reduced.

- Broken and damaged relationships may follow in the wake of bereavement, where not only the absence of the deceased has to be accommodated but new roles established in relation to the living. Changes in residence may bring the loss of many longstanding social contacts and friendships and the evolutionary movements in family living bring the exits and entrances of many people.
- Old age may bring a decline in physical and/or mental health, with short term illness and the onset of chronic conditions being characteristic. Accompanying these changes may be many adjustments to changed body image and physical functioning.
- Retirement is a time of changed economic circumstance and this may incur some element of disadvantage, lower income and inappropriate housing producing comparative or real poverty.
- The impact of unrealized aspirations is likely to be especially poignant for older people, who may be confronted with the ultimate reality of disappointments in relationships, and youthful dreams will also be part of what has to be grieved.

In all of these areas the significance of the loss to the older person has to be appraised, as well as the extent to which physical, emotional, social and/or spiritual well-being has been affected by the loss. Where primary sources of stability are lost (for example, spouse, home, physical mobility, etc.) then the impact will be greater than with more peripheral losses. However, while the examples given would be readily seen by the outside observer as significant, it should be recognized that some losses produce profound grief because they are significant to the person but are not necessarily seen as such by other people (for example, the death of a friend or a pet, the loss of a possession that has sentimental value, etc.). Sensitive attention to the 'meaning' of this loss and an understanding of the extent of the 'attachment', within the life of an individual, is crucial to making an effective response.

Current losses, either major or minor, can serve to reawaken unresolved grief from the past. This can be another situation in which there may appear to be a mismatch between current events and the reactions to them (for example, a miscarriage of 45 years ago may be part of what is mourned when an elderly widow is hospitalized and reminded, in the fear and loneliness of the experience, of emotions that were suppressed long ago).

GRIEF: A FACILITY

Grief is a complex psychosocial facility to accommodate loss. It is not a process of disintegration but one of reappraisal and adjustment and for older people faced by many losses grief will be a significant element within their experience. It is important to recognize that the 'stages' of grief are not discrete or time limited, but that they identify some of the significant aspects of psychosocial reality:

- denial and disbelief: a process of protection from the full impact of the loss;
- pain and distress: a process of identifying and expressing the emotions of guilt, anger, etc;
- partial accommodation of the loss: a process of making sense of experience, often accompanied by depression;
- acceptance of the consequences of loss: a process of integrating the past and investing in the future.

The response of denial is a feature of the early stages of grief, where the psyche would be overwhelmed with the reality of the loss if there were not a mechanism to hold its significance at bay temporarily. In older people, denial may be manifest in a number of ways including a deterioration in mental health, no concessions to new circumstances, a resistance to a new lifestyle and a preoccupation with the past (this may also be a feature of long term memory being more efficient than short term memory). The forcefulness of emotions may be seen most overtly in those who, for example, following a stroke have less capacity to control responses such as crying. For others, a lifetime of being controlled and not revealing feelings can produce behaviour which masks the real origin of distress, for example, being 'difficult', being obsessional, pestering about the past, etc.

For the carer, the disruptive or uncooperative elements of this behaviour will be problematic, especially if it has been interpreted as criticism and dissatisfaction with the care being offered. The apathy and withdrawal which is part of the depressed reaction to loss is most easily recognized but induces a feeling of helplessness in the carer. This may result in carers backing away and so isolating the elderly person, or trying to 'jolly' them along. Either response will fail to give the recognition to the grieving person and heighten their sense of loss.

The increase in loss and bereavement is no less painful because it is timely. It is perhaps the fancy of youth that the predictable losses of older people are somehow more bearable than the (tragic) losses at earlier stages of life. The ending of significant relationships, changed body functioning and altered social circumstances, after decades of established patterns and routines in life, carries its own trauma. 'Nothing left to live for', 'He just went to pieces when she died' – these are often the realities for older people, not the philosophical dismissal of 'a good innings', 'a peaceful death after a long life' which our grief-denying culture projects on to the situation.

FACING DEATH

One particular loss which is confronted in old age is that of one's own death. In one study (Littlewood, 1990) bereaved people were interviewed and relatively few under 45 had considered death or dying, while relatively few over 65 had not.

Reflection on this life event, in common with the assimilation and acceptance of other losses, will require an ability to make sense of experience. The capacity to do this may derive from a religious or philosophic view, which explains life and suggests purposes within life and death.

> Yet by death, by illness, by poverty, or by the voice of duty, we must learn, each one of us, that the world was not made for us, and that, however beautiful may be the things we crave, fate may nevertheless forbid them. It is part of courage, when misfortune comes, to bear without repining the ruin of our hopes, to turn away our thoughts from vain regrets. This degree of submission to Power is not only just and right; it is the very gate of wisdom.
>
> (*Russell*, 1976)

> How shall you find it [the secret of death] unless you seek it in the heart of life?
>
> (*Gibran*, 1972)

Making such views, or the many other religious or philosophical perspectives, one's own or arriving at a more individualistic sense of meaning is most creatively achieved with external support: the listening ear of a grandchild, discussion with contemporaries or dialogue with a priest. This can help to externalize and achieve clarity in the face of the internal struggle.

The final stage of integrating the past and investing in the future may not be possible where persistent losses, problematic resolutions and declining physical and emotional capacities hinder the process of accommodating multiple change and loss (Kubler-Ross, 1973).

CARER'S DILEMMAS

The participation of others in adjustments to change which an older person has to make brings its own difficulties. For relatives the griefs, perhaps of an ageing parent, bring attendant griefs to the children. 'I lost the mother I knew when she became deeply depressed after father's death' – the words of a daughter who is grieving the loss of father and mother and additionally identifying with the physical and emotional suffering of her mother. Watching the suffering of those who have supported us and cared for us in the past is especially difficult.

The social adjustment to changing roles demands a high degree of awareness and sensitivity. Part of the social consequence of loss is that the world of relationships is changed and for an elderly person it may be a very rapidly shifting reality. Relationships which have evolved and contained certainty now have to be renegotiated. However, it can feel alien to have to express one's needs to people with whom there has been a longstanding pattern of social engagement which has not included overt discussion of emotional and social needs. For example, the elderly widower whose past relationship with his children has been passive, as his wife was the agent of family communication, will feel very isolated in his bereavement, not only on account of his wife's death but with the loss of the link that she made with his wider social network. If that link is to be restored, conscious energy has to be put into establishing a new pattern.

Conflict and pain from earlier stages in a relationship may make carers ambivalent about offering support to an elderly relative. The dilemmas are likely to be great for an adult daughter caring for a sick or dying father who abused her in her childhood. Similarly for a daughter-in-law caring for her husband's parents who showed disapproval of her in the early days of her marriage, there may be strains and pressures. Finding ways of disengaging from past conflict will determine the extent to which carer and cared for will feel comfortable in their complementary roles.

This is a situation where counselling and support, perhaps group support, may benefit the carer. Resolving emotional conflict in a relationship can liberate the energy needed to care effectively. Where this resolution has not occurred during the lifetime of the elderly person, bereavement counselling can offer retrospective relationship counselling, which can be beneficial to the carer.

Balancing a range of responsibilities can be problematic both to family and professional carers. The middle-aged son who is heavily engaged in the demands of career and family may have little time to give to a bereaved relative. The busy social worker, caught in the compromise of being agent of public provision and agent of the best interest of her client, will carry much anxiety about limited facilities and restricted time available for elderly people. The 'hit and run' scenario is a familiar one where the carer's own sense of helplessness is translated into strictly time limited engagement with older people. So the victim status of those with a range of needs associated with loss will be compounded by social isolation. Small wonder that the dehumanizing and prescriptive reality of much provision for older people can leave carer and cared for in a combative state of victim against victim.

Time for choosing may seem to be past for most people in the later stages of their life. Limited human capacity and limited social provision is compounded by the tendency for carers to be prescriptive in their caring. The complexity of role reversal in families, when children become parent to their parent, is fraught with difficulty, not least the acting out of past unsatisfactory relationships.

COUNSELLING: '...BURN AND RAVE AT CLOSE OF DAY'

Counselling is a helping process which aims to help people to understand themselves and their situation better and consequently to modify aspects of feeling, thinking and/or acting which currently cause discomfort/distress/pain. Clearly, within the context of grief, there is much to be done to restore the psychological and social balance which has been disturbed by loss.

The growth of counselling is to be both welcomed and questioned; welcomed on account of the sensitive skill base which has become available as a strand throughout the caring professions, but questioned as a practice concept which might contribute to the de-skilling of lay carers, thus furthering the process which marginalizes human need to specialist corners of care. The balance of care expressed by relatives, voluntary groups and professional carers must be constantly appraised against the need to maintain the fullest measure of humanity that is possible.

In the face of grief what is the expression of the fullest measure of humanity for an older person? It can be:

- to listen and accept the repetition and apparently regressive aspects of grief (the many times told 'story' of the loss and the dependency which may accompany mourning);
- to facilitate a re-evaluation of relationships which have been lost through death or changed by other life events;
- to facilitate an exploration of future life choices – relationships, roles, lifestyle, etc;

- to foster a positive self-image in the face of losses which have removed key sources of recognition and affirmation for the individual;
- to maintain an objectivity that does not allow the helplessness of the older person to obscure the realities of their value or the possibilities that exist for them.

The person-centred model of counselling, based on the work of Carl Rogers, with its emphasis on the client's phenomenological world is particularly appropriate for work with older people. Here the measure of humanity, the valuing and enabling of another, is described in terms of three core conditions offered by the counsellor/carer:

- genuineness;
- acceptance (of the client and her/his situation);
- empathy (felt and communicated to the client).

This produces the climate in which psychosocial pain can be expressed and new directions explored. It is that enabling process which Shakespeare recognized as essential:

> Give sorrow words: the grief that does not speak
> Whispers the o'er-fraught heart, and bids it break
>
> (*Macbeth*)

Worden (1990) describes four tasks for bereaved people, which will equally apply in adjusting to other losses:

1. to accept the loss;
2. to experience the pain of grief;
3. to adjust to life without the deceased (or other person or object);
4. to withdraw energy from the past and invest in other relationships (and life objectives).

This framework allows for the significant psychological and social consequences of loss to be addressed. However, the resolution of grief is a lengthy process and in practice one is likely to see, with older people, a persistent struggle around the first three tasks, with little capacity to move into a totally satisfying new phase of life. Problems of complete recovery from the multiple losses of old age should not deter carers from recognizing the need to acknowledge the pains and fears of grief. These objectives may be explored also in group support contexts and indeed where residential accommodation is the unit of care, residents will need to be given permission to look at group and individual losses.

At its best counselling, or modes of care which incorporate counselling principles, can offer a new capacity to handle life's losses. The rage against the dying of the light is acknowledged and transformed into an acceptance of it.

CONCLUSION

The patterns of loss and change encountered throughout life may have provided a resourcefulness to meet the 'dying of the light' and its many endings with integrity and creativity. Alternatively, negative psychosocial experience may leave only the 'rage' of powerlessness to echo to the losses of old age. Describing and understanding these realities is the prelude to creating an environment which acknowledges the profundity of loss experiences and the vigour of emotional reaction to accommodate them. Counselling suggests both techniques and approaches which, in valuing the individual, assist in the painful orientation to the realities of growing older.

The challenge for us all is to accept the rage against the dying of the light, seeing within it the normal manifestation of the grieving energy which is part of life. An energy which can be helped to find creative fulfilment is the light that remains.

Note: This chapter is a shortened version of an article of the same title which first appeared in the *Journal of Educational Gerontology* of October 1992.

See also comments on burial by Nyanguru in Chapter 9.

PART ELEVEN
Training

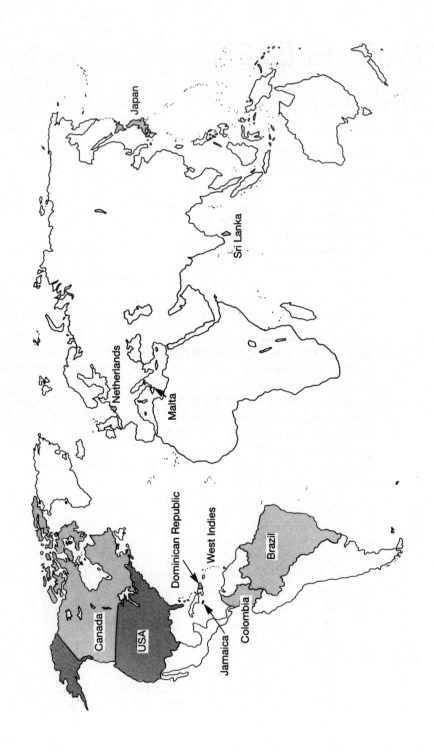

Training for elder care 36

Towards a Caribbean regional training system at the University of the West Indies

Denise Eldemire

The Caribbean, a group of islands whose inhabitants are mainly English speaking although Spanish and Dutch are also spoken, has been experiencing over the past ten to 20 years an ageing of its population. Two aspects of ageing are being seen: both individual ageing as an increase of life expectancy and population ageing as an increase in actual number of aged. These ageing changes are being experienced at a time of decreasing fertility and consequent decrease in family size with shifting contributions to the dependency ratio. They are also occurring at a time of great economic change.

As the population ages, new areas of interest and concern emerge. Two of these emerging concerns have been the care of frail or dependent elderly and the maintenance of optimum health according to the World Health Organization (WHO) definition, i.e. including social, economic and spiritual well-being, of independent elderly within the community. It is an accepted fact for both economic and social reasons that community based programmes are better than institutional care.

Elderly people are unique and individual and while not a homogeneous group with uniform needs, they do have special needs which differ from those of the younger and middle aged population and which need to be addressed at community level.

As societies undergo development and the processes of urbanization, industrialization, increasing participation of women in the workforce, economic hardship and structural adjustment, there has been an influence on family life and composition including attitudes towards the care of the elderly. The rising cost of health care for the aged is placing an increasing burden on the family and on society.

Furthermore, when the aged lose their physical prowess, their earning capacity and their companions (through death), an increasing responsibility to support such persons falls upon the family, relatives and friends. Where such support systems are not available, the burden is often passed on to the community.

Fortunately, with the marked improvement in health care now potentially available, it may be possible in some cases to postpone the incapacities of old age and to allow the elderly to remain physically, mentally and emotionally active well into their 70s and 80s. The more fortunate elderly, if employed and productive, may not prove to be a severe burden to the family, community or country until very late in life.

In developing countries where jobs are hard to come by in the first place, interesting philosophical, sociological and perhaps moral questions will arise with respect to whether the youth or the elderly should have priority to jobs which are such scarce and precious commodities and there will be challenges to design and implement strategies and programmes.

POLICY BACKGROUND

Following the World Assembly on Ageing in Vienna in 1982, six recommendations on training and education were included in the International Plan of Action on Ageing adopted by the General Assembly of the United Nations. Also, one (No. 7) of the 18 recommendations on health and nutrition is devoted to training.

In 1984, the Caribbean Health Ministers considered the elderly as a specific group for the first time, recommended that the meeting consider the elderly as a special group with special needs and endorsed the recommendations of Vienna. The Panamerican Health Organization (PAHO) in its Regional Programme has also started training initiatives in the region but these have been confined to Latin America.

A study group of Caribbean experts, meeting in Kingston in 1988, also made specific recommendations about training needs:

- development of retirement preparatory programmes;
- adequate training of all personnel involved in care of the elderly;
- programmes need to be directed at changing attitudes and not restricted to providing information and/or service;
- research to be extended.

The training programme is therefore very solidly supported by national and international policy statements.

Community based carers are of very varied disciplines in our countries, ranging from close family members to friends and neighbours, to trained social workers and they play a vital role in supporting elderly persons. However, until this training programme there was no programme offered for these persons to educate them on the ageing process and the special or unique characteristics of elderly persons. This was identified as a major problem by the carers in four community based surveys including one national survey.

Once the need for a practical basic training programme was recognized, the question which had to be addressed was: what institution would be most appropriate to develop and offer such a course? The University of the West Indies (UWI) was identified as being most suitable.

The UWI was chosen for two reasons. It is the training institution serving all the territories of the region and hence the course would be widely available. Secondly the University has a long tradition of being involved with non-degree programmes being offered to community based workers, the longest being the four month social work course which has been offered for some years. The very multidisciplinary nature and different levels of courses offered in the University make it a very appropriate place for integrated efforts in gerontological training.

The Department of Social and Preventive Medicine, which had previously developed a four month course for community health aides, was an ideal department to develop the course because of its experience, its community base and its community workers. Also the department was already involved in elderly programmes as some of its staff, with others, had started a non-governmental voluntary agency, HelpAge Jamaica, working with elderly persons and affiliated to HelpAge International and therefore in touch with other age care organizations in the region. In addition, the project director has had years of experience working with the elderly and teaching gerontology and geriatrics.

The project document stated that the objective of the three year project is to develop a four month training course at the University of the West Indies to offer training to carers of elderly people working at the community level.

SPECIFIC FEATURES OF CARING FOR ELDERS

Care of the elderly differs in important ways from the management of problems in other groups of people, whether paediatric, disabled or poor. First, ageing and its associated limitations are normal and are encountered by community workers themselves as they age. Few other health or social care areas have such personal significance.

Secondly, when considering health care, care of the elderly is different from disease prevention or treatment at younger ages. The health workers' satisfaction is often derived from their contribution to maintaining or improving the function and independence of the elderly rather than from dramatic restoration to 'full health'. Unless this difference is recognized and attended to in training, health workers are liable to feel professional frustration in caring for the elderly. Expectations, attitudes and tasks must be adjusted accordingly.

Thirdly, care of the elderly, perhaps more than any other type of care, is interdisciplinary. Team work is essential to ensure that medical services, nursing care and social domestic services complement one another in maintaining optimum quality of physical and psychological life, whether in institutions or in the community. Effective team work depends largely on health workers' awareness of and respect for one another's tasks, but there are certain team skills which can be learned, for example, those concerned with management, coordination, leadership, supervision, delegation and evaluation of team performance. However, these can be acquired only by practice under supervision.

A fundamental principle in the care of elderly people is to enable them to lead independent lives in their own homes and communities for as long as possible. There is every reason why this should be possible, since many elderly people, particularly those below the age of 75, are not much different in physical and mental capacity than they were in their 50s.

However, in many cases elderly people enter residential care for socio-economic reasons (lack of income, substandard housing, lack of an immediate carer) rather than because of failing health. To prevent this there is a need for a programme of community support services to enable the elderly to continue to be sustained in familiar surroundings.

THE TRAINING PROGRAMME

PARTICIPANTS

The training aims to reach community based carers of elderly people from both the private and public sectors. Among those initially targeted are home visitors and public health nurses working with the elderly in the community, staff of the National Council for the Aged, staff of day care facilities, social officers, poor relief officers, individuals such as family members with a concern for the care of older people. The programme aims to give training in all aspects of basic health and social care of elderly people including basic home nursing care. In addition, the programme seeks to give practical guidance on the establishment of caring facilities and the organization of voluntary groups for age care.

The participants accepted should already have had practical experience in the age care field and the course draws extensively on their expertise (for example, in the development of approaches such as case study work). All participants can read and write and preference is given to mature students who have, by their record of community based activities, demonstrated an interest in age care work. Social workers and those involved in Government programmes (such as the Food Programme) are eligible. Some participants are drawn from among the large number of voluntary organizers of small scale care projects in their countries.

SYLLABUS

The training programme staff identified ten basic objectives for the course and then worked with a training consultant to develop an appropriate course based on modules. Each module is complete in itself and forms the potential basis for short courses or a longer course for residential carers. The objectives are to develop the following skills:

1. an awareness and understanding of the needs of elderly people;
2. an understanding of the rationale of a specialized service reaching elderly people;
3. an ability to organize a support service to elderly people on the basis of a rational needs analysis;
4. basic nursing skills in care of an elderly person;
5. an ability to help elderly people to develop self-care skills;
6. basic skills in rehabilitation;
7. an ability to utilize family and community care resources;
8. recording and reporting methods;
9. self-evaluation skills;
10. good communication skills enhancing relations with elderly people and their carers.

COURSE CONTENT

The course will cover three broad areas:
1. knowledge of the principles of age care;
2. age welfare promotion and care;
3. organizational management.

Module A: The need of elderly people in the Caribbean

On completion of this module, participants will have an understanding and awareness of the needs of elderly people in the Caribbean.

Module B: Home care skills and rehabilitation

On completion of this module, participants must be able to perform basic skills in home care and rehabilitation

Module C: Self-care skills among the elderly

On completion of this module, participants must be able to help elderly people to develop self-care skills.

Module D: Family and community care resources

On completion of this module, participants will be able to utilize family and community care resources.

Module E: The development of interpersonal skills

On completion of this module, participants must be able to demonstrate a minimum level of interpersonal skills in the management of their relationships with elderly people and their carers.

Module F: Self-evaluation skills

On completion of this module, participants must know how to perform and respond to self-evaluation exercises.

Module G: Meetings, reports and recommendations

On completion of this module, participants must be able to produce effective reports and recommendations.

Module H: Field work and practicals

On completion of this module, participants will have put into practice all the material and principles taught in this course. It will consist completely of field work and practicals.

COURSE STRUCTURE

The course is intended to be run over four months, for approximately 15 participants with at least seven other territories in the Caribbean participating. The pilot course was run with six participants from Jamaica.

The methodology used in teaching was a mixture of theoretical and practical sessions. The practical sessions included discussions with elderly persons, visits to social and health related agencies both government and non-government, assignment to a family to identify strengths and weaknesses and case studies to work on. In addition, role playing was a vital part of the teaching methodology, such as blindfolding the participants while teaching how the blind cross roads.

The theoretical lectures provided basic information on ageing and the needs of elderly people and the lectures aim to relate theory to practice, the aim being to enhance the participant's practice of care rather than simply to increase theoretical knowledge.

The pilot course was extensively evaluated by the lecturers, the caring officers and the students initially and then reviewed by the training consultant who initially helped design the course. The evaluations did not result in any major changes and were useful in that they led to the design of a student manual to supplement the instructors manual for the next course.

COURSE ADMINISTRATION

The course was run by the project officer (a university lecturer) and a training officer. Experts in the field were used for specific lectures and financial management was by the administrator of the department offering the course. The training consultant visited four times and materials were sent back to him for review as they were written.

Each module had a coordinator who identified the appropriate person to teach and they worked with the training officer to ensure that materials were collected from the lecture from which to make appropriate overheads and handouts for the next group of participants.

The initial plan for the training programme covers five years so as to ensure continuity and to facilitate evaluation.

Year one includes:

- identifying and linking with key organizations and individuals in the region who would act as information resources in planning the course;
- a detailed analysis of needs and development of content for the initial course;
- holding of pilot course in conjunction with UWI academic departments;
- evaluation.

Year two covers:

- follow-up with participants in the initial course to evaluate effectiveness of training in modifying practice;
- planning and implementation of second course;
- evaluation and preparation for Year Three.

Year three passes on to:

- implementation of course;
- development of distance learning component through UWI network;
- research into further related training courses and preparation of feasibility study for a permanent training facility within the region.

Years four and five should achieve:

- implementation of course;
- implementation of new initiatives.

In summary, therefore, a practical training programme in elder care has been presented. It represents a joint effort between several organizations and individual persons. The course is particularly for community based persons caring for elderly persons and does not rely on First World well-developed technology and expertise. It does rely on a few committed caring people with a working knowledge of gerontology and can be replicated in local villages and communities wherever there are elderly people, their families and carers.

Bridging the patient – practitioner gulf 37

Interdisciplinary training in relationships in Porto Alegre, Brazil

Aloyzio and Valderes Robinson Achutti

As in many countries, there is evidence of a difference of attitude and comprehension between medical practitioners and elderly patients in Brazil. The course on 'Health Promotion and Protection III' has evolved a strategy to rectify this.

Brazil is a large country which already has a great number of elderly people needing care and support from one discipline or another. United Nations estimates suggested that whilst in 1950 Brazil already had 2.25 million inhabitants over 60 years of age, by 1990 the total would be 10.5 million (about equal to the UK total) and by 2050 could well rise to about 34 million. It was also calculated that by 1990 the average male Brazilian aged 60 would have a life expectancy of another 19.65 years (the highest in South America), whilst the female Brazilian could expect another 22.58 years of life.

These figures underline the need for efficient geriatric and gerontological services in this rapidly developing country where, until relatively recently, these services have been seen as of low priority. The patient–practitioner gulf could also be exacerbated by the fact that many elderly people were born and brought up in remote regions with few if any formal medical services, but have now moved to an urban area. There an encounter with a highly specialized geriatrician, surrounded by some display of modern technology, can be a frightening experience for a former rural peasant.

A NEW TRAINING APPROACH

More than 15 years ago a new method was introduced into the curriculum of the School of Medicine at the Federal University of Rio Grande do Sul, in Porto Alegre. This was an interdisciplinary module called 'Family Follow-up' which aimed to put students, from the beginning of their studies, into contact with people living in poor settlements (*favelas*) on the periphery of the city. Three years ago, this became a central task of the course 'Promotion and Protection of Health' in the field of the elderly. The elder focus complemented two other segments concentrating on mother and infant and on schoolchildren and adolescents. The elder focus, under the chairmanship of Professor Aloyzio Achutti, adopted five nursing homes with 100 residents of average age of 75. The students, who would be in regular contact with the elders, had an average age of 20 and the tutorial staff of between 50 and 60.

As the course developed other practitioner schools were drawn into the idea, including the course of Occupational Therapy at another university and the Programme of Health to the Elder of the State Department of Health. Since 1991 we have also included students from the Department of Internal Medicine, the Department of Social Psychology and the University of the Third Age. The gulf-bridging concept therefore ranges across the spectrum of health disciplines into social work.

The inclusion of the University of the Third Age is important as those older students do not participate as 'guinea pigs' but as a liaison and monitoring group to facilitate the contacts between 20-year-olds and 75-year-olds.

Both students and elderly subjects were alerted to the fact that the students did not visit in the simple roles of additional assistant physicians. The normal medical and health service to the subjects would be maintained. The 'gulf-bridging' students' task would be that, over a six months period, each student would pay a weekly visit to the same selected elder to try primarily to establish understanding and a friendly relationship. Obviously such a relationship would also enable the elder to have better access to appropriate services as well.

There were minimum and maximum assumptions. The maximum was that the programme would explore the riches of a specialized professional-cum-human relationship for the benefit both of the professions as a whole and of the patient community. The minimum assumption was that, even if this did not improve specialist services, it would be at least a worthwhile exercise in human relationships. In fact, from these visits there sprang a plethora of questions, suggestions, proposals and actual projects of action which the course directors encouraged and helped to carry out.

As questions and subjects arose during the visits the course was moulded into a theme system covering the following concepts:

• heredity – genetic, social and cultural;
• actual opportunities for health and development;
• risk factors and disease;

- death and dying;
- depression and dementia;
- submission and domination (practitioner v. patient);
- interventions for promotion and protection of health;
- organization of groups to work against health risks.

As optional activities the visiting students were also invited to participate in some research projects, which gave the students additional impetus in the visits. Small groups of students work with an orienting professor (often from another sub-specialty) in several research projects which need not be limited to the duration of the course but have extended access through the course. These projects cover a wide range of subjects, such as cardiorespiratory resuscitation, urinary infection in older women, self-medication and drugs in use, dementia and depression, organization of self-health groups, etc.

The older students from the University of the Third Age not only have a liaison function in the programme but are required to report back on the attitudes and progress of the visiting students. A report back is also obtained from the visited subjects themselves. However, some of the most vivid insights into the worth of the programme come from students' own reports. It must be borne in mind that the majority of students may well originate from social strata and sub-cultures very different to the visited subjects and having very little initial mutual comprehension.

PRE-TEST PRECONCEPTIONS

A pre-test is given to students. This consists of a blank piece of paper on which they are required to say what thoughts arise in their mind around the themes of 'elder' and 'ageing' and what are their own expectations from the exercise. This paper then remains as their attitudinal start point and the measure of their subsequent progress in understanding.

In the 1991 pre-test, only two students mentioned that in the future they too would be elderly, recognizing the continuing process of ageing. Half of the students cited decay, fragility, functional limitations and so on as being dominant attributes of the elder, with remarks such as 'the body is no longer the same and cannot accompany the mind'.

In this pre-test profile of the elderly, several negative physical and psychological traits were delineated, with a number of students taking care to state that these were not their own objective judgements but 'received knowledge' from general societal attitudes. The following aspects, among others, were mentioned: white hairs, muscular mass decay, locomotion problems, wrinkles, dependency on the family, incapacity, loneliness, abandonment, depression, sorrow, frustration.

Although the main feature was the predominance of negative over positive concepts, a few of the latter were stated, including experience, knowledge, wisdom, maturity, developed capacity to interpret the world.

The idea of diseased old age loomed large, especially degenerative diseases as a sequel to lifestyles and as accidents of the culture and environment. One student wrote, 'I remember my grandparents whom I knew as always ill, and they died while I was a child'.

Also included in these initial remarks were the need for a special type of care for elders as distinct from care for younger people and also the extent of blame apportioned to society, the family and the State for the treatment which old people received. But one student commented, 'To tell the truth I never before considered how one ages or what it is to be old'.

POST-TEST COMMENTS

It is naturally fascinating to compare pre-test papers with a post-test examination of the same student cohort. It was specifically required that frustrations and problems should be reported as well as successes in changes of concept about ageing. The comments were so varied, specific and personal that it is difficult to prepare a statistical synthesis, but the common factor was the general satisfaction with having established a friendly bilateral relationship which, to many of them at the beginning, had been unbelievable. 'Before, I avoided contact with old people because I was afraid to touch on their sentiments.' The sensitizing process revealed its efficacy in the anxiety of most of the students about the impact that the end of their relationship would have on the visited elder, even though a new student might be taking their place at the beginning of the next academic year.

Whilst a number of students reported changes in their own concepts of elders, a somewhat lesser number agreed with the student who wrote, 'My original concept of the elder did not change, but I acquired a different perception on how to establish a relationship with an older person, something which is only possible through practice'.

Among 'gratifying experiences' could be counted the following:

- When the lady I accompanied said to me that I was the daughter God never gave her;
- I liked to arrive there and to see that I was awaited with anxiety, offering me coffee, cakes, etc. Many times I was obliged to accept, seeing that this was so important to her;
- I felt myself useful just helping Mrs X. to adapt herself to the new life in a nursing home;
- When Mrs H. said to me 'Say to your mother you now have two mothers, she and me'.

'Frustrating experiences' were faithfully recorded:

- Not to be able to remove from the mind of Mrs E. some ideas such as to be old is bad, and old people aren't worth anything;
- To see that what we were doing was very little, considering the extent of the necessities of these persons;
- Verifying that she did not receive a visit from relatives either over Christmas or at the New Year;
- The accelerated demential process of Mrs A.; so frequently she told me the same stories and sometimes she seems to go into fantasies;
- The bad smell emanating from Mrs D.... shameful and a lack of respect to her in the way of deficient care.

Some of the perceptions arising from the relationships of these inexperienced students with elders, who were often in a confused state, are worthy of wider circulation and study. Among these would be the comments:

- It is necessary that society not only shows compassion (sometimes with hypocrisy) about the limitations of the elderly, but should try to appreciate fully their qualities;
- The only aspect I changed in my previous perception was that the elder, even those living in nursing homes and being needy persons, still have a future and hope;
- Mrs M. is illiterate but one day she started to recite poems from Brazilian classics. She learned by heart, only by listening. Although unable to read, and suffering from symptoms of ageing, she is of very high intelligence;
- It is difficult for the elder to accept himself as he is, but even more difficult is not to be able to live the ageing process in his own way... tied to misconceptions, myths...;
- We must let the elder be, in their own manner, the elder they did not want to be;
- I became sad with the idea of separating. We agreed to continue contact by telephone and I promised to visit her again. But to say 'goodbye' is something one cannot avoid.

There have been difficulties in implementing this idea, not least in the coordinating of diverse disciplines. We are working people from several schools, visiting the same nursing homes. From time to time the tutorial staff from different schools have coordinating meetings. But, due to timetables and other curricular duties, it is impossible to have a regular meeting of students where the whole group can interact.

NEW STRATEGIES PLANNED

Next year we shall develop two strategies, firstly to extend the use of University of the Third Age students, and secondly to videotape seminars and student exchanges as material for further discussion. In the last year 16 students from the new University of the Third Age accompanied the activities of the students on the course.

The Third Age programme is an initiative of our Department of Social Psychology. They have what is still an experimental curriculum offered to about 150 persons of more than 50 years of age. This group, mainly women, have to give one afternoon a week to traditional classes, but beyond that they can take up a number of optional practical activities. This provides an excellent pool for extending our project beyond nursing homes to include a number of non-institutionalized elders within their own homes.

We have now been able to enlist this group of elders on a formal basis for two ongoing functions. The first is, as previously, to act as individual liaison between course students and the visited elders, but also developing a sub-project of themselves (the University of the Third Age people) evaluating the impact upon the subjects of the students' visits. Their second involvement will be to draw into the programme suitable subjects among external elders living locally in their own homes.

RECOMMENDATIONS

We here in the Federal University of Rio Grande do Sul have come to certain conclusions about the scheme and would particularly mention the following:

- Older persons in nursing homes can draw great benefit from the systematic visiting of younger people.
- The experience of provoked human relationships between university students and older people – not only as a solely professional encounter – outside the ward or consulting room is necessary for an adequate professional training.
- Among these students, before they are subjected to educational procedures which may cause distortion to these qualities, there is already present a capacity to understand the elderly, an ability to make effective transactions with distant generations and across social classes, an interest in the ageing process and the reaction to it, a sense of compassion and a certain creativity of thought.
- Students benefit from an interdisciplinary approach.
- The interest of sub-specialists can be obtained without monetary investments through the development of mutually advantageous research lines into ageing, which also secondarily can bring rich benefit to the cohorts studied.
- Elderly people are becoming a social stratum interesting to academics in the social and health care approach because they are needy, they

are a group of specific size and, in general, they are as yet unexploited as objects of genuine scientific investigation.

All that has been described emanated from a professorial chair in a medical department but the approach throughout has been intensely practical, personal, individual, free of imposed restrictions and driven on an interdisciplinary basis. It follows that the scheme could have originated from any other sub-specialty with an interest in ageing. Equally the training is applicable to any activity, professional or lay, salaried or voluntary, which has daily dealings with elderly people.

The concept of considering bilateral personal relationships with individual elders as an appropriate and recognized segment of sound studies and training is therefore recommended to all agencies who are concerned for the greater welfare of the many more old people who will need care, support and opportunities in the future.

Training, retraining and reintegration 38

Areas of training activities for elderly programmes (Canada, Colombia, Dominican Republic, Malta, Netherlands, Japan, Sri Lanka, Thailand, USA)

Ken Tout

This brief survey covers three areas of training which are of vital importance in the development of ageing programmes. It does not include 'pure education' undertaken by older persons for their own pleasure or intellectual benefit. Nor does it include 'public education' in the way of awareness campaigns. Rather is it related to training which teaches and develops specific skills. The three areas are:

1. training or retraining of older workers where either the worker wishes to continue working after an imposed retirement age barrier or a person needs to vary skills as his/her ability to cope with the current work load diminishes;
2. training of carers in skills needed for work with the elderly, in this case the term 'carer' covering an entire range of roles from family or volunteer carer in the home through geriatric practitioners and on to the training of trainers;
3. the use of older persons themselves in a training or educating capacity, either for their peers or for young groups.

RETRAINING OLDER WORKERS

In regard to the first area of activity, one expert with a role strategically located for an international view has written:

> Good recommendations continue to outpace good practice as far as employment-related training for older persons in industrialized countries is concerned. Despite the proven track record of older workers and accumulating evidence that age is not a handicap to continued learning, employers remain reluctant to invest resources in their training and retraining.
>
> *(Nusberg, 1990)*

However, she is able to provide some examples of good practice. Japan has an excellent record compared to many other countries and 47% of companies with 5000 or more employees have training programmes for older people. Among smaller companies, of up to 99 employees, the figure is still 17%. The Fuji Photo Company offers all employees between 40 and 55 years of age a specially designed course with three components dealing respectively with technical skills, health and personal 'quality of life'.

A survey in the USA showed that workers of the 50–62 age group in 44% of cases looked for an update of current skills from training, whilst 33% wanted training in order to get a different job. At 63 and over the main preference was still for updating but in that age group some 31% did not desire further training as compared to 10% earlier.

The famous food outlet McDonald's has a scheme for training and placing persons over 55 years of age as being reliable labour. There is a four week training period averaging from 15 to 20 hours a week in all aspects of the work. The firm also offers the advantage of flexible working hours.

On coming to the age of 50, employees of IBM Netherlands are given the opportunity to discuss their continuing career and any training which might be needed in order to diversify. This policy was first prompted by high disability drop-out of outdoor manual workers and women working on assembly lines. The cost of disability benefits or early retirement was so high that it was found to be economic to offer training and relocation within the company at around 50 years of age. The company also offers to cover costs (up to 3000 guilders) of any specialist course which might be appropriate for an employee at this stage.

The provincial Government of Ontario in Canada has introduced a scheme called Transitions. This has the twofold objective of encouraging older unemployed workers to take up retraining for suitable re-employment and providing financial backing for individual workers to undergo such training. Up to 5000 Canadian dollars in training credits is available, either to pay costs which employers may incur for retraining workers re-entering the job market under this programme or to pay tuition costs for a worker taking up retraining at any public or private training institution recognised by the provincial Government.

Eligibility for entry to the programme is as follows. The entrant must:

- be 45 years of age or older;
- have experienced, within six months before application to the programme, termination of permanent employment resulting from an employer going out of business, closing or moving; termination of employment due to a shortage of work; or the failure of a self-operated business;
- have not, at the date of application, found comparable, permanent employment;
- be seeking to update existing skills or obtain new or replacement skills;
- be a resident of and entitled to work in the province of Ontario (Schulz, 1991).

TRAINING THE CARERS

Moving to the second field of activity, that of training carers, examples are given in Chapters 36 and 37 in more detail. If relatively more is done in developing countries by way of varied job training and retraining, as compared with the (obviously far greater volume) programmes still being evolved in 'The North', in 'The South' there is a relatively larger deficit of practical training for carers. I myself encountered the case of a fairly large developing country which, in the mid-1980s, had no single practitioner who had received any formal geriatric training.

Possibly the first highly organised and intensive volume programme for lower grade carers in ageing in a developing country of the middle grade took place in Sri Lanka. As at that time there was no training available for any carers who had actual contact with older people, HelpAge Sri Lanka targeted its course at a group of carer types, including social workers, therapists, home carers and organisers, as well as nurses.

The course was extensive and ranged from detail of domestic care chores in the home to practical nursing of the levels which might be expected to have frequent application in the case of older people. The course was designed by a qualified nurse trainer and, after some trial and evaluation, was produced in considerable detail in 12 modules. In this way a theme module might be selected for a short workshop and an intelligent organiser new to the material would have enough detail to teach and guide the elements of the module.

The course, which was an eminent success in Sri Lanka, was then transferred to Thailand with few adaptations and again was found to apply to local requirements. The modules, with other useful information, were then produced for general replication in similar countries by HelpAge International.

At about the same time the Colombian Pro Vida organization (as described in Chapter 39) was offering experience in its network of varied ageing activities in Bogotá to other interested agencies, both from the provinces of Colombia and from neighbouring countries. Most of the participants were from the voluntary sector but representatives from official services also attended. 'Crash courses' of three weeks to one month were arranged for groups of about a dozen persons who were as much observers as students. Courses tended to have a bias towards relevant themes such as income generation or intergenerational activities.

Space and staff were provided by Pro Vida under the programme title of CIGAL (Spanish acronym for International Gerontological Centre for Latin America). Training schools of Bogotá universities provided lecturers to teach alongside experienced Pro Vida staff in the didactic element of courses. But much of the course period was spent in observing and discussing in detail the various Pro Vida responses to the problems of an ageing population in a country experiencing migratory transition. For national students further more advanced and exhaustive courses were coordinated between Pro Vida and the collaborating universities on the academic campus.

The Malta Government, which had been instrumental in persuading the nations of the world to hold the World Assembly on Ageing in 1982, continued to play an innovative part in training. It combined with the United Nations Ageing Unit in Vienna to set up INIA (the International Institute on Ageing) in premises provided by the Malta Government.

The remit of the Institute includes that it 'shall provide training in gerontology at various levels to persons, particularly from developing countries, who hold positions as policy makers, planners, programme executives, educators, professionals and para-professionals dealing with problems in the field'. The Institute is able to call on the services of international teachers although much of the value of courses is found in the exchange of views and experiences among student groups which may represent, in one course, nations as varied as Argentina, Bangladesh, China, Saudi Arabia and, of course, Malta itself.

A MODEL COURSE

A particular short term training programme in income security for the elderly will demonstrate the type of training offered. The course was of 12 days duration and consisted of nine blocks plus an orientation, pre- and post-training evaluation by the students as well as staff, and opportunities to visit some of Malta's excellent services for the elderly.

The blocks were allocated as follows:

Block 1 (8 hours) General framework

Objectives and principles: challenges of an ageing population; various approaches to income security; need for variety of answers to hetero-geneous needs; problem solving and policy formulation and evaluation techniques; the 'contract' between generations; instruments and actors of policy.

Block 2 (16 hours) Current situation of elderly and future projections

Age, rural/urban, male/female breakdown; definitions; labour force distribution of elderly; health indicators; work cycles and retirement patterns; sources of income; benefits programmes; relative levels of poverty at different ages.

Block 3 (8 hours) Policy context of well-being and income security

Integration/coordination of policies; possible ways of ensuring adequate income; aspects to be harmonized (housing, health, labour, subsidized prices, etc.); immigrants, minorities and the destitute; transitional international economy.

Block 4 (4 hours) Assessing the needs of the elderly

Appropriate data; living arrangements; life cycles; 'objective' assessment, as from experts' judgements; 'subjective' assessment as from older persons' own perceptions; comparisons and criteria.

Block 5 (24 hours) Alternative approaches to providing income security

Classification of approaches (statutory/urban/cash, etc.); analysis of existing methods (universal benefit/provident funds/employer-sponsored/self-help, etc.); alternative methods of financing such schemes; systems of organization and administration; measures of adequacy; protection of benefits (inflation proof, etc); links to national development.

Block 6 (4 hours) Special needs of elderly women

Life cycles as workers; disadvantages; differences in retirement ages; life cycles as spouses, widows; left alone in rural areas; contradictions in provision of income security (home makers, disabled, divorced, etc); special role as caregivers.

Block 7 (8 hours) Emerging trends in changing environments

Demographic; role of women; increased education; urbanization; participation of older persons in formulating policies; social disintegration; public and private sector functions; flexible work systems; future economic growth to sustain social policy innovation and globalization of economy; increased flow of ideas and information.

Block 8 (4 hours) Communication skills

Demonstrations of; role play; use of audio-visual materials.

Block 9 (8 hours) Field experience

Site visits to relevant agencies in income security, such as Departments of Statistics, Social Policy, Social Security, Pensions; income generating projects locally. (More information on this and other courses is readily available from INIA.)

Evaluation of two rather different courses from the USA points to important lessons. A nine month training programme for occupational therapists in Philadelphia is structured on a three phase basis. The first concentrates for three months on health care needs of the elderly and their informal caregivers. There is a didactic component followed by a field experience period leading to a concluding seminar. The second phase involves working within an interdisciplinary care team. Finally there is a 'dissemination' phase during which the student has the opportunity to crystallize and consolidate the acquired knowledge and skills by preparing co-authored presentations (Gitlin and Corcoran, 1991).

The third phase is perhaps remarkable because it occupies four months out of the nine and enables the new student to 'disseminate an innovative service model to a wide audience'. However, perhaps even more notable for wider replication to other types of carers' courses is the second component of the first phase, which places the student alongside the informal caregiver. The student acts as temporary support and respite, but also feeds in fresh ideas for care. The informal but experienced caregiver is able to either explain any objections to a given idea or to share with the student a time of experimentation to the mutual advantage of student, caregiver and care receiver and also, if the idea is successful, for information to the wider audience.

In the field of dementia, a Cincinnati specialized Alzheimer's centre offers unique opportunities for students to have first-hand experience of personal dealings with patients. Emphasis is put on sharing the positive aspects of life as may be possible at specific stages of the disease, rather than attending only to negative manifestations. There is, of course, a classroom element and meetings with staff of the centre but it is in the 'clinical rotations' that students may profit most and where the significant lessons for replication may be found (Gilster and McCracken, 1991).

Students are given a basic grounding in aspects such as mission statements, staff training, individualised care planning, environmental design, behavioural management, cognitive assessments and life enhancement for persons with dementia. Then they move into the rotation system which sees them each working with impaired residents of the centre for short periods. It is an essential requirement that students should not be diverted into chores like bedmaking or meal preparation.

At first it was considered that these clinical rotations should be an experience open only to graduate students; that students would only benefit by observing and working with patients for long periods; and that patients might be disturbed or scared by having contact with too many students on too frequent a rotation. Protection of the patient was a first priority.

Over a course of time it was seen that all these assumptions were to some degree or other incorrect. Students of lower grade than graduate were equally able to benefit. Short rotation periods showed no disadvantage to the students' progress in acquiring skills. Patients were in no way disturbed by having more frequent visits from a greater profusion of unknown students. In fact the patients responded positively. The experience of shock or fear tended to be found in the students rather than in the patients. It was the students who needed 'protection' in the form of careful preparation as to what they might encounter.

ELDERS AS EDUCATORS

The third area of activity to be mentioned here concerns the use of elderly persons as trainers and educators. A number of projects have shown the ability of elderly people to pass on practical skills to younger cohorts, today as in ancient times. More than one instance of this exists in West African countries. In each case local traditional trades, particularly in ceramics, had been allowed to lapse in days when new mass-produced modern imports were proving cheaper and more popular than slow process, handcrafted articles from the traditional lathe or potter's wheel. However, when inflation made the imported goods inaccessible, retired craftsmen were recruited to revive the local industries, working alongside young apprentices.

A more direct experiment in elder pedagogy is under way in the Dominican Republic and utilizes similar experiences from 'older' countries to the north. With the title 'LinkAges' the project operates in two phases, using older people as an educational resource in schools and arranging specific activities to help children towards an accurate and positive view of ageing and the elderly.

The programme centres on a rural area near the border with Haiti and removed from the Republic's main urban concentrations. Retired teachers and elderly community leaders are used to teach children, initially in the 3–6 year old group. This is because research suggests that most children may have adopted their attitudes towards the elderly by eight years of age and by 12 years of age the attitudes become difficult to change.

In addition to teaching and joining in intergenerational activities with the schoolchildren, the elderly participants will also help to revise school curricula, positively to include material which will enhance understanding and conversely to eliminate prejudice and elements which might promote undesirable attitudes. The dangers of stereotypes of ageing make it important also to watch for any injurious influence on children emanating from the press, television, political statements or family behaviour.

For the youngest children the 'gerontological' lessons will particularly feature older people in their roles as valuable participants in agriculture, child care, health matters and the preservation of traditional culture. It is expected that the long term development of the programme will enable the production of suitably tested teaching materials which can be widely replicated.

Twenty three communities with a population of over 10 000 people were surveyed in order to set up 20 early childhood programmes with elderly teachers in local schools. The survey showed that 10% of the total local population is between the strategic ages of three and six, whilst 11% of the population is aged 60 and more – as against a national average of 6%. The average age of the instructors is 58, although the preference is to offer opportunities to the oldest who are able to participate.

The project, which is sponsored by the international agency SSM*BRIDGES, could eventually offer to other interested agencies:

1. an intergenerational early childhood education curriculum that has proved successful in a developing country;
2. a programme to train older adults in developing countries to serve as early education instructors;
3. intergenerational education materials;
4. a guide and training manual for organizing early childhood develop-ment projects featuring older persons as resources (Fernandez-Pereiro and Sanchez-Ayendez, 1992).

The Dominican Republic venture in some ways resembles the Generations Together Senior Citizen School Volunteer Program of Pittsburg, Pennsylvania, USA. There elders work in schools for an average of four hours weekly throughout the school year. Students involved are of all grades from 1 to 12, as distinct from the pre-school approach of the LinkAges project.

An evaluation of three years' data from the Generations Together programme was carried out and in its methodology emphasizes a number of points which should be considered in evaluation of this and similar types of enterprises, including:

1. the problem areas that typically emerge during the development of intergenerational programmes;
2. the elements of intergenerational programmes that enhance their probability of success;
3. the components of intergenerational programmes that can be replicated and how this replication can occur;
4. the persons in a community who can benefit from intergenerational programmes and the nature of these benefits;
5. the role of systems and agencies in the creation of successful intergenerational programmes;
6. the societal issues that can be addressed through intergenerational programmes (Bocian and Newman, 1989).

During the evaluation process the perceptions of both elders and children were tested as to programme outcome. Among elders 87% noted an increase in feeling needed; 71% recorded greater openness to new ideas; and 69% experienced an improvement in their attitude towards children and youths. Responding, the younger group showed 97% success in academic progress; 84% with a greater appreciation of life skills and 95% declaring better and happier attitudes towards older persons.

It might be hazarded in conclusion that a similar evaluation of outcome with younger teachers might not have been so complimentary.

PART TWELVE
Organizational

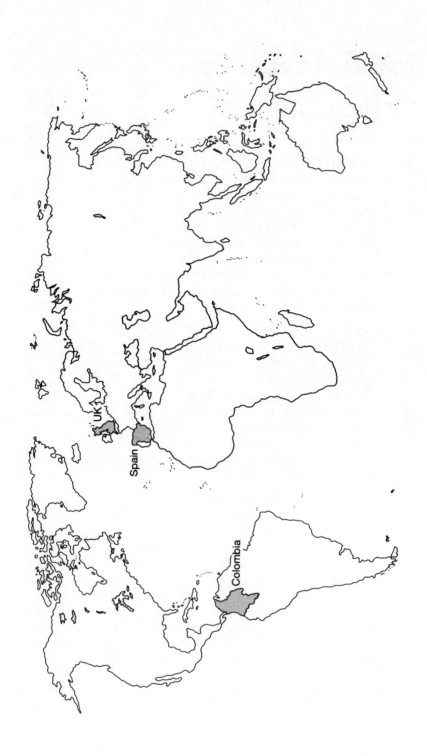

Genesis of a care organization 39

The Development of Pro Vida, Colombia

Eduardo Garcia Jacome

Colombia is a typical example of a country that is undergoing the three 'ageing' factors which may eventually precipitate a socio-economic crisis in some developing countries as well as in older industrialized societies. These are a dramatic fall in both mortality and fertility rates – leading to an increase in the proportion of elderly people within the population – and continuing rampant migrationary movements.

Since 1970 the number of over-60s has increased every year, with a corresponding increase in the percentage of elderly. That 'dependency ratio' is estimated to rise from 4.3% in 1970 to 11% in 2020. This would mean, in gross numbers, an increase in over-60s from less than 1 million in 1970 to about 5.5 million in 2020. At the same time the rural to urban migration has been so great as to totally reverse the statistics over a 50 year period. Whereas the country's urban population had been 37% against 63% in rural areas, by the end of the 1980s the urban areas had 63% and the rural areas only 37%.

There were two other significant factors about migration. As in most migration patterns it was mainly the younger people who migrated, often leaving older people without immediate support in a depopulated and distant rural area. Also in Colombia much migration was by step; that is to say that the migrant did not always move directly from the home rural base to a new permanent urban setting. Often it was a move from rural hinterland to a larger town and then on, some time later, to the capital Bogotá. In Bogotá there might be two or three brief periods of residence in varying shanty conditions before a permanent settlement, if that ever occurred. This made it difficult for older people to follow in the migratory steps of younger relatives.

However, many elderly people found their way to less affluent areas of Bogotá and, due to many factors including lack of housing, had to live alone in the most distressed circumstances or as members of family groups in inadequate dwellings and under great stress of poverty.

FIRST ACTIVITIES

Pro Vida's focus on the problems of these elders began as a relatively modest endeavour by a small group of concerned citizens who took it upon themselves to go visiting local old people's homes, bringing a little cheer to persons living out their days in abysmal conditions. One of the homes visited was a dilapidated old building in which some 750 elderly or mentally handicapped persons were offered shelter by a small, devoted but totally inadequate team of some 13 nuns, many of them also elderly. The visiting group included a number of professionals with practical skills who did their best to ameliorate conditions, although at first these efforts were at what might be called the 'odd job level'.

The visitors identified some 30 similar homes, usually run under impossible circumstances by dedicated nuns, but having little or no stable income provision or other resources. Most of them had no access to medical attention, for instance. It might be said in defence of the authorities of the day that, because traditionally in Colombia the old person was looked after by the extended family system and because the increasing abandonment of elders was a new phenomenon, there had never been, in earlier periods, need for a Government structured welfare state type of provision for the elderly.

The group's experience in the home for 750 persons contributed much to thinking about development of the visiting programme. Clearly the very welcome operation of arriving with a few parcels of 'goodies' from time to time, or the fixing of some dripping taps, was not likely to improve the situation of literally thousands of inmates of such establishments. At the same time, in spite of the poor conditions, the nuns held long waiting lists of older people wishing to come into the homes as being preferable to a life of abandonment on the inner streets or in the outer shanties. The fact that the 'laundry' for the 750 inmates consisted of three old zinc baths with no running water caused the visitors to plan long and hard.

The first concept was that a request to raise funds for a commercial sized washing machine for the home would not be viable if it merely led to another 30 requests from another 30 homes for similar, and evidently urgently needed, equipment. So, it was argued, why not attempt to obtain an even larger machine which could handle the laundry for all the homes? And, having obtained such equipment, why not use it also for external commercial work as a continuing fundraiser for allied projects? And if a commercial laundry could be contemplated, why not also a bakery on a similar scale, so that a regular supply of basic food could be guaranteed to institutions whose financial problems were so acute that from time to time even the daily bread was in short supply? And could not such an enterprise employ some elderly people who were not yet ready for entering an institution but who had no sure resource of income or family support?

A MAJOR PROJECT

Pro Vida's own survey showed that only about 20% of elderly persons had an assured source of income such as a retirement pension (mainly for government employees or members of multinational enterprises) or significant life savings. So attention needed to be paid to the problems of those elderly who were not yet admitted to the lesser evils of one of the residential institutions. But the capital cost would be substantial by local standards and there were, as yet, no sufficient means of raising large sums of money within the country. Could international funding be sought and secured?

In the event, international funders were attracted initially by the bakery proposal rather than the more material laundry concept. So a project was planned and edited to ensure that the bakery would have truly 'developmental' implications. It was to fund itself for posterity by producing and selling high class bread and confectionery to retail customers coming in from the street. It was to employ directly a number of local elderly people. It was to donate half its considerable production to identified old people's centres. And it was still to make a revenue profit to provide modest funds for other projects envisaged.

Ambitious though the objectives might have appeared, the funds for implementation were raised, suitable premises were found and donated and equipment was installed with the advice of local master bakers who enthusiastically approved the scheme. An excellent publicity stroke was the launch of a 'Delicacies of Yesteryear' competition in which elderly inmates of the institutions were provided with the raw materials and the opportunity to produce confectionery 'such as Grandma used to make'. These recipes became very popular for housewives visiting the bakery which had been opened on a main avenue where no competition existed.

An attempt was made, in the interests of economy, to run the bakery entirely with a staff of willing volunteers. The same concept was used for the laundry which, over a period, had also been funded and in-augurated, again with a service both to the street and to needy insti-tutions. But there were problems with quality of production and with the complicated economics of donating 50% of the production outright, a principle which was strictly adhered to from the commencement of operations. After about 18 months it was realized that the employment of a fully qualified bakery manager would be more likely to achieve the high targets required. After the initial phase a profit was forthcoming and went to help fund a free medical and dental clinic upstairs from the bakery.

Meanwhile, the retail outlet of the bakery had become a prime centre for an awareness campaign aimed at shoppers who had not yet recog-nized the changing population profile of the nation or who had not yet realized the implications of the breakdown of the extended family system as the old age insurance of national elders. Although inter-national funding sources had been generous both with cash and skills, it was evident that an ongoing programme must have sufficient and stable support locally. The general public, the media and national and local authorities must be persuaded to turn their attention to this new phenomenon and its potential crisis implications.

The national Government had already legislated for a national council on ageing to be set up in the 1970s but this good intention had been buried under a weight of other urgent social and economic priorities. Approaches were made, at the highest level, securing goodwill from the President downwards to move towards a national programme but which would take time to plan and introduce. The original group of visitors had grown to a significant company of volunteers, trained and recog-nizable in their smart blue overalls. The group had found it necessary to use an alternative to the original association's registered name, *Asociacion Nacional de Establecimientos Privados de Asistencia al Anciano*, which was not the most convenient label for fundraising or for interviews with the impatient mass media. So *Pro Vida* ('For Life' – a longer and a better life) became the brief and easily remembered front name. And its bread (*pan*) was *Pan Vida*!

PUBLICITY BREAKTHROUGH

An early breakthrough came when persistent approaches to television stations produced a request for a personable elder to appear on a Christmas charity spot on a nationwide TV programme. An elderly man, who had suffered abandonment but become rehabilitated as a Pro Vida volunteer, told his story simply before the cameras and became a TV star overnight. Such was his impact that his 'slot' was repeated on various

TV programmes 240 times during that Christmas period, free of charge! Similar success was achieved with a short but professionally produced (by volunteers) Pro Vida film which the national distributors gave 'B' film treatment at cinemas throughout the country. Pro Vida had also formed its own concert party for the sole entertainment of elders and friends.

When a further aid grant was offered from international sources Pro Vida, again with an eye on publicity, asked for the purchase of a bus which would be available to all elderly people from the growing numbers of institutions and day activities sponsored. The bus, which would display awareness publicity posters, would be travelling all hours of every day on its compassionate missions, ranging from hospital visits to countryside picnics. Soon the vehicle was widely recognized by street junction policemen, other drivers and the general public who gave it VIP priority in the dense Bogotá traffic.

Another indirect route of awareness campaigning came through Pro Vida's recognition of the possible virtue of copying British systems which encouraged children in sponsored events to 'Help the Aged'. Youthful promoters went into local schools to teach about ageing. Events were arranged in which children successfully raised substantial amounts to sponsor new activities with the elderly. In many cases families of the children involved were able, through Pro Vida's promoters and the school teachers involved, to establish and foster relationships with abandoned grannies and grandads from the shanty areas.

The success of the schools campaign enabled Pro Vida to negotiate with the Ministry of Education so that final year school pupils could elect to take part of their Social Studies syllabus studying and working with Pro Vida. In addition to studying aspects of ageing the pupils were guided in setting up educational projects by which groups of the pupils visited old people's centres and gave presentations, illustrated by their own visual aids and role play, to elderly people, particularly in aspects of urban life of which recent rural immigrants could be ignorant.

TRAINING DEVELOPMENTS

The training aspect of Pro Vida had grown from initial brief training of local volunteers to the stage where a training centre was prepared. In typical Pro Vida extempore fashion this commenced with the simple roofing over of the patio until such times as the success of the practical operation justified more sophisticated surroundings. The centre was ambitiously given a name including the word 'international', its acronym being CIGAL. Within two years interested planners and volunteers from more than a dozen other Latin American countries were attending CIGAL courses to study Pro Vida projects and the means by which these could be replicated in their own countries. Pro Vida staff travelled to the same countries for follow-up consultancy as new national programmes were launched. (Pro Vida Peru and Pro Vida Bolivia are among other age care agencies which have evolved during this period of mutual co-operation, each as independent national entities.)

It was only a step from the growing CIGAL activities to negotiation with universities and training colleges so that Pro Vida's unique expertise could be allied to academic methodology both in the training of professional carers and in new opportunities for the elderly themselves to study at academic levels. Much earlier, initially in a corner of a room above the bakery, Pro Vida had initiated basic training for elderly people with no income. This included literacy, ceramics, embroidery and a number of useful crafts which would bring some income to the worker after a two to three month course. Instruction was also given in small business management and, in a number of cases, an elderly person returned to an impoverished family of younger relatives to set up a family business with the elder as the founder and expert.

The growing public awareness of the nation's ageing problems and the recognition of Pro Vida's initiatives not only produced income support but also increasing calls for care for new cases of abandoned elderly. Trained social workers were on hand, assisted by volunteer professionals such as doctors and dentists giving their time as possible, to deal with an almost frightening increase in care demands. Eventually the operation which had grown from a handful of willing visitors now found itself with nearly 30 000 cases on its books.

MORE INNOVATIONS

To cope with the demands, new publicity and funding ideas were evolved such as the previously locally unknown idea of substituting a charity donation for flowers as a funeral tribute. Now through the *Canitas* (Silver Hairs) scheme bereaved younger relatives can 'adopt' an abandoned grandparent for a year, providing a quota to purchase groceries or medicines or leisure opportunities for that person. In the *Canitas* scheme help has been forthcoming from supermarkets and credit card agencies as well as obituary column editors.

Whilst the main focus of migration and of Pro Vida's projects has been on the capital city of Bogotá, time and resources have been found to help local groups in other regions to begin their own similar programmes, often with innovative ideas such as the local group which has obtained a municipal monopoly on recycling of waste, with elders as staff. The least emphasis in Pro Vida's programmes has been on the establishment of any kind of bureaucracy, although in some functions – as was found with the bakery – expert service is invaluable, particularly in such areas as editing of good publicity, including videos and training manuals.

Pro Vida's standing was consolidated in official and public esteem when, in a national volcano eruption catastrophe, it was early on the spot and was entrusted with the rehabilitation of all elderly victims. This merited donation of a fully equipped ambulance from HelpAge, to use both in future emergencies and in the continuing disasters of endemic poverty.

NOT WITHOUT PROBLEMS

The record of Pro Vida reads like a story of unfailing success. In fact, as with any organization launching into operations without precedent, there have been problems along the way. Possibly one of the most painful problems was related to the efforts to use well-meaning but untrained volunteers for tasks which really required a professional approach. In some cases this was successful – as, for instance, with an accountant giving spare time to work on accounting or a volunteer architect able to assist with minor projects. In other cases the use of a professional from day one would have shortened the initial phases of a project and, in the long term, would have been an economic investment.

Whilst generous support came from a number of countries overseas, it was sometimes necessary to subordinate local plans or judgements to the understandable preconditions of international aid and, on occasion, this could lead to a more complicated and less effective development. In the replication of practical projects it became clear that even a transfer of any idea to another smaller city or to a nearby rural area could require serious consideration and adaptation of the original format.

Another extremely sensitive area is the sense of ownership of a low key project by the particular group of carers and organizers, so that a developing larger organization, of which that 'grassroots' is a part, may appear to become an unwelcome 'Big Brother' agency wishing to interfere in the smaller considerations. To an extent Pro Vida has been able to identify and cope with such problems because it has retained a core of the original type of volunteer in its hierarchy. It has not surrendered the higher direction of the agency to impersonal if efficient external executives who might not have the same vision of commitment, which last factor is seen as being the essence of the organization's success:

personal commitment, by young and old alike, to the welfare of those less fortunate.

Note: Pro Vida is not related in any way to the Catholic Church's 'Pro Vida' anti-abortion campaign which is well known in some Latin countries.

An integrated strategy

40

Outline of the Plan Gerontologico for integrated services in Spain

Rafael Pineda Soria

The most developed countries have discovered in recent years that one of the outstanding sociological phenomena is the ageing of the population. Spain is not excluded from this problem. Our country, too, is ageing and at an accelerating pace.

It is sufficient to say that in 1960 persons over 65 represented only 8.2% of our population whilst by 1990 the same group accounted for 13%. Translating this data into absolute numbers, I have to say that from 2.5 million persons over 65 registered in 1960, there are now already more than 5 million Spanish people over that age. Looking to the future, projections of population foresee that by the year 2000 there will be more than 6 million Spaniards of that age group, representing 15% of our population.

At the same time in Spain, as in other surrounding countries, there has taken place in these last years a profound social transformation. Among other factors we must note that the traditional function of the family is in a state of profound revolution; that the classic role of the woman is going through a serious mutation due to her incorporation into the work force; and that personal autonomy has increased. Such phenomena have their positive side, but it cannot be denied that they have developed some negative consequences for older people, including loneliness, isolation and social marginalization.

In fact the needs and demands of those over 65 have been deduced from sociological research carried out recently. This gives evidence that, in a majority of cases, the level of welfare which has been achieved in recent times has not reached those citizens of higher ages, those who with much sacrifice and difficulty have contributed to reaching the very level of development which Spain enjoys today. An analysis of the resources which our society was offering to senior citizens manifested both the scarcity of these and also the lack of quality, whilst there were regional disadvantages in their distribution.

It is also necessary to add that the texts of recommendations from international bodies require that we should adapt the standards and levels of protection of older people in line with the rest of the European Community. This aspiration is also a requirement of our own Constitution. Finally, such targets were an election undertaking of the party elevated to Government in October 1989 – *Partido Socialista Obrero Español.*

The needs of older persons in Spain are mainly reflected in the following factors in synthesis:

- Whilst there is the guarantee of a pension for every older person in Spain, there are still elders whose income is insufficient. At October 1991 the average monthly retirement pension was 55 445 pesetas and the widows' pension averaged 34 618 pesetas.
- Whilst there is universal access for old people to medical and pharmaceutical services, more than half those over 65 were presenting untreated symptoms, in spite of repeated visits to doctors.
- More than a million elderly people, largely women, live alone and that isolation often signifies marginalization and want.
- 65% of people own their own dwellings but many of those are very ancient and with little comfort, lacking modern conveniences, with 11% situated on upper floors in buildings lacking lifts.
- About 92% of older people are either illiterate or have attended only primary school. Few go to public events, nearly 90% never go to a cinema and 49% never go on holiday.
- Relations with younger relatives are often rare as younger people become absorbed in their own careers, whilst, now that they have so much time available, it seems that nobody requires anything of those retired people who have so much to give.

Retirement, which could be the era of joy and the period of opportunities, has been converted for many into a difficult journey...to nowhere!

CONTRIBUTIONS TO THE GERONTOLOGICAL PLAN

In putting together the Plan account has been taken of the demographic and sociological research already referred to, as have the deliberations of experts in the various relevant subjects. Also taken into account, for it could not be otherwise, were the recommendations formulated by the representative associations of older people. Others who contributed included responsible politicians from the Autonomies (the autonomous regions into which Spain is divided), the conference of social affairs, the interterritorial council of the National Health System, non-governmental organizations, trade unions and other experts concerned.

THE CONTENT OF THE GERONTOLOGICAL PLAN

The Plan, which seeks to make an integrated response to the various aspects and matters related to the ageing population, is set out in five major areas of operation: pensions, health and medical attention, Social Services, leisure and culture, and activities.

In respect to pensions, although these have increased significantly in recent years, the prime preoccupation of older people continues to be with economic security. The Plan aims to increase pensions in line with increases in cost of living, guaranteeing the non-contributory pension right to all citizens over 65 and establishing an additional element for pensioners over 80 who have insufficient income and who need the aid of third parties because of their own incapacity.

On health and medical attention, the Plan will stimulate the promotion of health and the prevention of illnesses and accidents, encouraging physical exercise and healthy habits and improving primary health care both at health centres and in people's own homes. Adequate hospital attention will be guaranteed with a strengthening of the geriatric potential and rehabilitative medicine. Professional training will be an essential part of these programmes.

As to Social Services, the Plan seeks to establish a full network promoting, above all, those services which enable the elder to remain in his own environment. In Spain, in the recent past, almost all the Social Services budget for the elderly has been used in the construction of centres, mainly day centres and residences. There has been scarce development of more innovative ideas of the kind which relate to integration within the community. One of these, service of assistance to domicile, whose advantages have been demonstrated beyond doubt in the experience of developed European countries, has not yet been extended sufficiently in Spain. And again it is necessary to underline the inequalities of the distribution of services territorially.

Of the remainder of community services, such as adaptations to housing, family support, day stays in centres and so on, these have not yet reached the stage of replication which would be desirable.

So whilst a general and considerable extension of the Social Services network is anticipated in the Plan, the following are seen as priorities:

- adaptation of dwellings as may be required;
- reservation of sheltered places in new housing projects;
- a considerable network of special accommodation such as individual apartments or small groups where security, assistance and fellowship can be found;
- the development of a programme in which older persons would be welcomed into voluntary family units.

Culture and leisure figure in the Gerontological Plan so that retirement might be the beginning of a process full of possibilities of personal self-realization. Hence:

- ways would be opened up to enable our elderly to enjoy our historic and cultural heritage, have full access to holidays, visits to seasides, excursions, cultural exchanges at both national and international levels, recreational activities and personal educational opportunities;
- to safeguard popular traditions, there would be full opportunities for traditional craft activities and the elderly would be encouraged to pass on their own cultural wealth (to others).

Society needs the productivity of all its members, and especially the experience of the elders, to continue building a world of more solidarity in which all – children, youth, adults and all ages – would live together and be mutually enriched in their human and social intercourse.

So that the participation of the elderly in the life of society shall be more than an expression of desire, the Plan will encourage associative movements and create organisms, such as councils of the elderly, which will contribute their experience and defend their interests in the development and continuity of the Plan.

GENERAL OBJECTIVES OF THE GERONTOLOGICAL PLAN

In order to give an overall vision of the aims of the Plan, which may have been lost in the extensive detail above, the following are cited as general objectives:

1. To develop a system of non-contributory allowances to persons over 65 who have insufficient economic resources and to offer an addition to the pension for persons of 80 who have lost their personal autonomy.
2. To improve the minimum pension and the remainder of the contributory pensions, guaranteeing their revaluation automatically in line with the cost of living index.

3. To promote health for the elderly and improve their physical, psychological and social well-being.

4. To guarantee within the general framework of the National Health System services of prevention and attention to the elder by means of adequate primary and hospital services.

5. To obtain delivery of community primary health services to the elderly, within a sectoral framework for which there will be designed a blueprint of areas within which these services can be integrated and coordinated.

6. To strengthen administrative structures for the development, coordination and equitable distribution of resources, so that there will be permanent study, investigation and planning on themes related to ageing and the elderly.

7. To offer appropriate Social Services which will respond to the needs of senior citizens, emphasizing above all those which empower personal autonomy, permanence within the domicile and continued living within the habitual community.

8. To increase the awareness within society of the social impact of the ageing of the population and the psychophysical characteristics of older people, together with an appreciation and recognition of the value and contribution to the cultural heritage of those who have attained advanced ages, as well as the participation and incorporation of these latter in social policy.

9. To facilitate the access of older persons to cultural opportunities and foster among them a creative use of leisure and free time, in order to improve their quality of life and their ability to consider themselves of use.

10. To extend the concept of democratic participation so that society incorporates in reality the elderly members and that these may be involved in reality in social life.

A CHALLENGE FOR THE DECADE OF THE 1990s

This is the challenge that we have marked out for ourselves up to the year 2000. It is projected that the Plan should develop throughout the decade, for whilst there are some measures whose execution can be realized at a specific date, others need to be developed over a long period of time which could hardly be less than the period which now distances us from the horizon of the year 2000.

It is expected that, in the course of these ten years, it will be feasible to close the door on a social policy which was aimed at the elderly but distinguished by institutionalization and by a concept of the retiree as socially useless. On the other hand, the period should see a stimulus and definitive commitment to a new concept in which the pattern will be of an integrated service directed towards a group of citizens who do not have to accept lesser rights just because they have counted more years.

Ensuring optimum services

41

The importance and methodology of evaluation

Andrew Sixsmith (UK)

The information provided by evaluation is essential if we are to ensure that the best possible services are provided, that financial resources are used effectively and that the quality of life of frail older people is enhanced. This chapter will outline the basic principles of evaluation and also point to some of the problems encountered by researchers.

The central theme is that evaluation is a 'worldly' science (Cook and Shadish, 1986) and that conventional scientific approaches are not always appropriate to the political and practical realities within which research is conducted.

WHY EVALUATE?

Broadly speaking, evaluation is a matter of judging the effectiveness and efficiency of a service or scheme. This involves defining what the objectives are and determining whether these are being attained. Evaluation provides information on which decision makers and service managers can act to ensure the best possible service. The ultimate aim is to improve standards and to enhance the well-being of the service users.

These are commendable aims and it would seem only natural that any organization that claims to provide 'care' for people should ask themselves questions such as 'Are we providing a good service?' or 'Where could we improve things?' and so on. But if we look at the appalling history of the way frail, elderly people have been treated by health and welfare services, then it is difficult to believe that these kinds of questions ever crossed the minds of professional caregivers.

As well as the need to do more evaluation, it is also important that the evaluation is done properly. Unless appropriate concepts and methods are used by competent personnel, then evaluation will be ineffective in improving services. Indeed, there is a very significant danger that inadequate evaluation will hide the real problems. The example of residential care in the UK is illuminating on this issue. Independent evaluation of private sector care homes by the statutory health and welfare agencies became a legal requirement under the 1984 Registered Homes Act. However, the scope of the act meant that this system of inspection was limited to basic issues such as health and safety or staffing levels within homes. Despite statutory evaluation, 'horror stories' in the press and from pressure groups about degrading and inhuman care practice remain depressingly frequent. There are signs that the situation is improving and recent initiatives by the Social Services Inspectorate and the Department of Health show a commitment to ensuring adequate quality assurance procedures that emphasize the quality of life within residential homes.

Evaluation is more than just monitoring standards of care. It is about providing information that will enable decision makers to maximize the benefits of a service and make the best use of limited resources. This kind of strategic information is becoming ever more crucial as both the demand for care and financial pressures increase. The fragmentation of the care economy further emphasizes the need for evaluation. Funding agencies and purchasing organizations operating at 'arms length' from care providers need to be aware of whether money is being spent effectively. This moves us from the 'what' questions of service monitoring to the 'how' and 'why' questions of analytical research.

WHAT IS EVALUATION?

Having dealt with the need to evaluate, I will now go on to outline some of the basic approaches. A number of components may be involved (Rossi *et al.*, 1979).

DEFINITION OF OBJECTIVES

Any service has some aims, desired goals or a policy. The actual service is the way of achieving these objectives and will involve the specification of clients, procedures and estimates of costs/resources. It is important that the evaluation should define these aims as precisely as possible. Key questions include:

- What is the demand for the service?
- Who are the clients?

- Is the service/intervention appropriate to the problem?
- What are the links with other services?

SERVICE OPERATION

A fundamental part of any evaluation is to ascertain whether a service or scheme is doing what it says it is doing. Key questions include:

- Is it operating in line with stated procedures?
- Is it reaching the target population?
- Is it integrated with other services?

SERVICE IMPACT

Impact assessment measures the extent to which a service or scheme causes change. Impact studies tend to be rigorous in a scientific sense, so that conclusions are persuasive. Control groups, matched samples and before and after studies are key approaches in the classic experimental approach. Less demanding and less resource intensive approaches may include expert judgements or client self-ratings. Key questions include:

- Is the service effective in achieving its intended goals?
- Are there unintended effects?
- Does the service make a difference to the quality of life of the client?

ECONOMIC CONSIDERATIONS

The financial aspects of a service are a central part of evaluation research. Concern is with value for money: the costs of service delivery and relative efficiency relating costs to outcomes. Cost benefit analysis and cost effectiveness analysis are basic approaches. Key questions include:

- What are the costs involved in delivering services to clients?
- Is the programme efficient compared with alternatives?
- Do the benefits warrant the incurred costs?
- What is the long term viability of the scheme?

EXPLANATION AND UNDERSTANDING

It is important that the evaluator understands the processes that occur within a service agency or scheme. The evaluator has somehow to look 'inside' the scheme in order to explain why problems are occurring or why a scheme is successful. Such insight affords greater confidence in drawing conclusions, making recommendations and applying results elsewhere. Key questions include:

- What are the main factors that have determined the relative success or failure of the scheme?
- Is the scheme characterized by cohesiveness or conflict?
- Are outcomes dependent on factors outside the control of the service?

Taken together, these would represent a comprehensive evaluation. It is important to stress that the different components should not be taken in isolation from one another. For example, a service may be highly effective, but may be too expensive. Evaluation is also an incremental activity. For example, if a scheme is not having the desired impact, then there may be no need to assess its economic consequences.

Results of applied social research and service evaluations have often had only a minimal impact on the problems that they have addressed (Cook and Shadish, 1986). However rigorous and thorough the research might be, it is of little value if it is not effective in facilitating change. Three issues need to be considered: the political reality within which decision making is located; the practical reality of implementing change; and the constraints under which the research is undertaken.

EVALUATION IN ITS POLITICAL CONTEXT

The results of research are often 'lost' within the political world of day-to-day decision making. Results can be conveniently forgotten or suppressed if they do not fit in with current aims and practices, while the recommendations of the research project may be shelved if they are not easily implemented within the current decision making context. Worst of all, the research may have asked the wrong questions and have provided information that is of limited relevance to the service providers.

Dryzek suggests that even where serious attempts have been made to synthesize evaluation within a problem solving framework, this may be unfruitful if:

> ...it fails to address its political setting. This setting in turn is defined by the value orientations of actors, the constraints upon these actors, and the structure of their reasoning.
>
> (Dryzek, 1982)

In an attempt to overcome this problem, there has been an increasing emphasis on providing information that is 'usable knowledge' within a given decision making context. A researcher must be aware of the potential opportunities and constraints that may affect the implementation of recommendations and the way the evaluation information is used. It is important to identify those decision makers who will use the information that the evaluation produces. The evaluator works with these people to develop relevant evaluation questions from which appropriate methods of data collection and analysis develop. Effective information has a number of characteristics:

1. Content is precisely defined: the information is focused on a specific problem and the concern is with tangible results and opportunity for implementation.
2. Appropriate information: the information is presented in a form that is appropriate to the decision making context. The presentation has to be understandable and convincing to all those involved in the decision making process.
3. Research duration: the turn-round time between problem definition and the production of information should be minimal. Information is usually needed 'yesterday', a requirement that should be taken seriously. Conventional approaches are usually concerned with methodological rigour, rather than the client's need for rapid results.
4. Involving decision makers: the information should derive from procedures in which decision makers are involved from the start. This affords a commitment to the outcomes of the research.
5. Scope: the problem domain and solutions should be of a manageable size. Weick (1984) suggests that it is important to produce visible changes by addressing manageable problems with small scale solutions. Taken together, a series of 'small wins' may be more effective in the long run than tackling all problems at once.

This 'action research' involves a reorientation in the way research is carried out. Instead of intellectual domination, the role of the researcher is to take seriously the expertise of all actors and to articulate their beliefs and understandings.

THE PRACTICALITIES OF CHANGE

Evaluation differs from academic research in that the aim is not just to describe or explain things, but to facilitate change. The political factors described above are important constraints on this process. However, as well as these, an evaluator must be aware of the day-to-day practicalities of introducing change within any organization. For instance:

CONSTRAINTS ON IMPLEMENTATION

Once a new service or scheme has been set up, it often becomes impractical to change or dismantle it. This is particularly the case where large amounts of resources are tied up in capital expenditure, such as building and equipment. Thus, the notion of evaluation as providing feedback that can be directly applied to decision making may not always be feasible.

THE PROBLEM OF GENERALIZATION

A key problem is how research findings in one context can be translated into practice in other contexts. All schemes have unique characteristics. There is no guarantee that the same inputs in a different context will have the same results. McLaughlin (1985) points to several factors accounting for this:

- Outcomes are not just dependent on inputs, but also on the existing context.
- Local choices dominate outcomes. Local differences in resources, commitment, attitudes and so on will mean that similar schemes may have entirely different outcomes.
- Implementation is a developmental process. It is not just a matter of 'installation', but a process of learning new practices and skills and developing new norms and beliefs.
- Multiple goals are often involved. As well as formal goals, any scheme will involve many informal goals in practice. The specific mix will shape actual implementation.
- 'Street level' decisions are usually the most influential. Often, it is at the point where policy is turned into actual service or care provision that crucial decisions are made.

THE PSYCHOLOGY OF CHANGE

The underlying aim of evaluation is to improve services. This is done by eradicating bad practices, enhancing existing approaches and developing new ways of doing things. However, the results and recommendations of an evaluation have to be acted upon by real people with different hopes, desires, abilities, fears, etc. Clearly, the psychological processes that are involved in this are of crucial importance. If recommendations are too dramatic, then service providers may feel unable to cope with the required changes (Weick, 1984).

These practical considerations place considerable constraints on the direct translation of research findings into care practice. Bearing this in mind, the objective of evaluation may be better seen as one of 'enlightenment' rather than one of 'implementation'.

THE RESEARCH PROCESS

A third area of concern lies in the actual design of the research. The practice of evaluation has developed primarily from an academic background, using traditional scientific approaches. However, the discussion so far has suggested that an evaluator has to consider factors that lie well outside the conventional view of research. For example, the notion of 'usable knowledge' would appear to compromise the ideal of a detached, objective and value-free scientific approach.

Traditionally, evaluation has adopted approaches and methods from pure research, where experimental, quantitative research designs have been dominant. However, the traditional experimental research design is often impractical within the time and resource constraints of an evaluation. For example, it may not be possible to use necessary research instruments or set up control groups. Cronbach (1986), arguing at a more conceptual level, also suggests that a blind adherence to 'hard' scientific approaches can even limit the progress of enquiry by undervaluing the insights and understanding that are characteristic of 'softer', hermeneutic approaches.

These considerations have prompted a move towards naturalistic approaches, such as participant observation, direct observation and open-ended interviews (Lincoln and Guba, 1985). The orientation is exploratory with an emphasis on insight into problems and processes within the research domain rather than establishing 'facts'.

Returning to the political and psychological contexts of evaluation, clients may expect 'hard', quantitative data and may feel uncomfortable with research designs based only on 'soft' qualitative data. Multimethod approaches that utilize a range of research instruments help to overcome these problems: both hard and soft data are produced, while a range of methods provides a 'triangulation' approach that increases confidence in the information that is produced.

EVALUATION AND SERVICES FOR THE ELDERLY

Here I would like to take a more specific perspective and look at evaluation of services for older people, to develop some conceptual, methodological and ethical issues that have not always been fully recognized or articulated by evaluators.

In recent years there has been an increasing emphasis on the measurement of service outputs as the criterion for judging the effectiveness of a service. One phrase which has become almost indispensable over the last decade is 'quality of life' (QOL). The welfare services that are provided for older people should actually have a positive effect on their wellbeing. However, despite the importance of the concept, there is very little consensus about what QOL means. Is it about happiness or life satisfaction or having some kind of meaning in life? Or is it a more limited concept, referring just to the basic living circumstances of a person?

The lack of definition is worrying. Without a better understanding of the nature and meaning of QOL, there is always a danger that the results of ill-conceived and misguided research will be translated into equally ill-conceived and misguided policies and practices (Sixsmith, 1993).

Even if these kinds of conceptual difficulties did not exist, there are also methodological problems facing evaluators. For example, people with dementia not only pose questions of what quality of life means, but also questions about how it can be measured. If a person is unable to communicate or understand simple questions, then the usual approach of asking them questions or administering life satisfaction scales is obviously inappropriate. Researchers have resorted to indirect methods such as observation or third party opinion in order to overcome this problem. This leads to further difficulties: can we infer inner states of mind and well-being from observable behaviour? Can we trust the opinions of others? Even with people whose mental faculties are intact there are still difficulties. In residential environments, the processes of socialization and institutionalization reduce the credibility of responses to a researcher's questions. Respondents may only have a limited awareness of alternative services and they may feel vulnerable and be unwilling to say anything that might be seen as criticism of the place in which they live.

Older people in general have often been seen to be very accepting of their situations despite the social inequalities, such as lower incomes and poorer housing conditions, that often accompany old age. Several factors may account for this (Sixsmith, 1993), such as low expectations or lack of information about rights and services. Research that fails to account for these factors will inevitably be a partial view and must surely limit the value of the whole exercise.

A last point takes us into the realm of ethics and questions about how and why evaluations should be conducted and particularly questions about the values implicit within research. I have already suggested that the ideal of value-free, objective research may not be entirely appropriate to the realities within which evaluation takes place. In order to provide 'usable knowledge' the evaluator may have to compromise scientific ideals and take on the role of an insider within an organization.

However, the notion of 'usable knowledge' does have drawbacks. Providing solutions that can be operationalized within a given decision making context may merely reinforce existing structures. Usable knowledge implies information that is geared to problems and solutions defined by decision makers, which may ultimately be of little relevance to important social problems (Cook and Shadish, 1986). For example, an evaluation might be able to show that a residential home provides good residential care for frail older people, but this says nothing about whether this is the best way of caring in the first place. In most cases, the solutions to problems are already defined and evaluation amounts to little more than finetuning and rubber stamping.

Whose values dominate? In whose interests do services really operate? Research is a practice that is undertaken by real people in a real world and is certainly not immune from the ageism that is inherent in society. Remaining scrupulously 'scientific' and methodologically 'correct' is insufficient if this only provides a partial and limited view of reality.

So how can these problems be overcome? Perhaps the solution lies in the recognition that evaluation is a very different animal to conventional research, requiring different approaches, techniques and perspectives. For example, Lincoln and Guba (1985) suggest a notion of authenticity to replace the scientific notion of research validity. This requires researchers to consider issues such as honesty, fairness, integrity, education and action rather than a mechanistic adherence to an academic science.

It is also important that research proceeds from a critical perspective, where the emphasis is on challenging appearances and accepted practices. Frail older people represent one of the most vulnerable and marginalized groups within society, a fact that is mirrored and reinforced by the way they have been treated within the caring services. Research needs to be about giving these people a voice and enabling them to exercise real power and control over their lives.

PART THIRTEEN
Women ageing

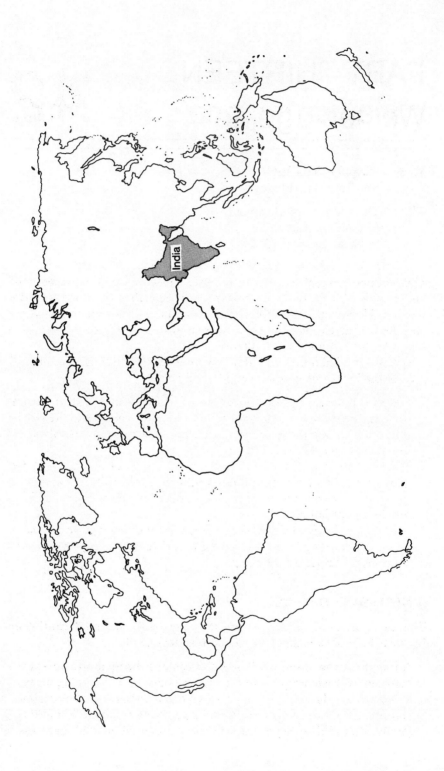

A woman's place? 42

Ken Tout (World view)

This volume has not sought consciously to differentiate between male and female elderly or to include projects specifically aimed at older women. However, it is appropriate to make mention of the need for specific consideration of elderly women although this could require a separate and complete work (Gibson, 1985).

Specific consideration of elderly women is justified on a number of counts, but just three might be mentioned here:

1. General interest in women's rights worldwide makes it important that the particular circumstances of elderly women should not be forgotten among many other considerations which may mainly affect women of younger generations.
2. Traditionally women have been the main carers for the incapacitated elderly of many cultures and the continued availability, or otherwise, of women carers will have a major effect on future planning for a greying population.
3. Demographically and socially, women are the majority sex in many ageing factors and could often be found to be the major sufferers from negative aspects of ageing.

A NECESSARY DEBATE

This is an area of debate where it is necessary to tread cautiously because, to quote a recent United Nations document:

An aggravating interface has, on occasions, been found to exist between 'women's rights' and 'family responsibilities' protagonists. Many women have been forced to a virtual surrender of all rights and opportunities in order to care for someone disabled within the family. Proposals of legislation to compel daughters or daughters-in-law to care for parents could provoke bitter conflict. On the other hand some assurance of understanding and sympathetic support for the proposed carer could produce more rapid and satisfactory solutions to individual family problems.

(Tout, 1992)

That document therefore proposes, as a part of overall strategy for care of the elderly, 'a Bill of Rights for carers, or clear policy statement of the relative rights of those who might be expected to render care within the family'. As a step towards such a definition of possibly conflicting rights, the proposal for an interim action was 'a conference of women representatives of various ages, of those who potentially may need care and those who potentially may have to care'.

Demographically there is no argument about the fact that, apart from a very few countries like Yemen and Qatar, older women outnumber men of the same age group, with the disparity tending to increase with age. One authoritative study, using 1988 data, quoted the increase with age in females per 100 of the older population for selected countries as follows:

- China – 50.6% at 65–69 years old, rising to 62.9% at age 80+
- Zimbabwe – 48.1% at 65–69, rising to 56% at 80+
- Brazil – 55% at 65–69, rising to 63.0% at 80+
- Turkey – 51.7% at 65–69, rising to 59.8% at 80+ (Kinsella, 1988)

The countries quoted here have been selected from a much wider range of countries in Kinsella.

Studies of matrimonial status produce extremely worrying results, taking into account the detrimental effect of widowhood on the elderly woman in many cultures. A crossnational study revealed such discrepancies as in urban Malaysia, with 85% of older males still married but 61% of older females widowed; in rural South Korea, with 82% of older males married but 55% of older females widowed; and rural Philippines, with 86% of older males married but 45% of older females widowed (Andrews *et al.*, 1986).

A commentary on this variation points out:

There are several reasons for the gender disparity in widowhood found in developed as well as developing societies. The most obvious factor is simply that women live longer on average than men. There is also a nearly universal tendency for women to marry men older than themselves, thereby compounding the likelihood of women outliving their spouses. Furthermore, widowed men are much more likely than widows to remarry... and the consensus of existing research is that the married fare better than the non-married on a number of dimensions...

(Kinsella, 1988)

Whilst the World Assembly on Aging of the United Nations, held in Vienna in 1982, was the first major international focus on ageing as a whole, a major focus on elderly women developed in 1985 in conjunction with the United Nations Conference for Women as the final meeting of the International Women's Decade. It was acknowledged that adequate information on the economic situation of older women worldwide was not possible to obtain as yet. However, many pertinent points were raised in the course of debate by participants from many different countries.

WORLDWIDE CONCERN

The document 'Conversations in Nairobi' records many of these points (Conable, 1986), of which the following are a selection:

- Young mothers appeared to be at odds with their mothers-in-law. They did not want the older women to spend time with their grandchildren because 'old mothers give children wrong ideas' (report from Japan).
- Today's emphasis on education has left the older and often illiterate Kenyans feeling useless and ignorant ... elderly are often left alone in villages without family assistance (Kenya).
- Older women ... experience tension when living with their children and grandchildren because of differences in values and lifestyles ... Yet they lack the financial resources to live independently and fear the loneliness implicit in living away from their families (South Korea).
- A major chain of stores went bankrupt and the employees, mostly older women ... were forced into early retirement. When the business was resumed ... the jobs were filled by younger inexperienced males. The women ... experienced depression and other psychological problems (Belgium).
- Employers often believe that older women workers can't learn ... another myth, that older workers have high records of absenteeism because of frequent illness ... that women work to secure funds for unnecessary purchases and therefore do not require reasonable wages (USA).

An African survey (Hampson, 1982) produced some almost frightening comments from older women who were just existing at the lowest economic stratum of life, comments which could certainly be reproduced from many other regions:

- My future life is very bleak and hard. I am useless and I think it would be much better if I died.
- In our African custom relations are supposed to look after one another but if the relations think one is too old, then life can be very lonely.
- I have nothing of my own. I left my home to others and I have to

squeeze myself into this tiny room.

- Today people no longer greet the elders; they even ambush and beat us old people.

At the other end of the economic spectrum there is firm data that comparative national prosperity does not necessarily 'percolate down' to older women of that society. An Australian cohort study states:

> The current generation of older Australian women is much more likely than older men to be living alone and to be living on very limited incomes. By all indicators of social need, older women are clearly disadvantaged ... superannuation schemes are designed to 'reward' loyal employees, and fit the traditional pattern of male working lives ... Without some attention to these issues, future generations of older women in Australia are likely to remain economically disadvantaged in old age.
>
> (*Rosenman and Winocur, 1990*)

Similar conclusions were reached in a study for the European Community. Looking at the experiences of older women in the 12 member states the report commented:

- It is not uncommon for over 10% of the women aged 55 and over to have never been married in the European community.
- In Germany ... 26% more women are in the lowest income group than men of the same age.
- Of the elderly population in the UK ... 78% of women are in the lowest income group.
- Evidence suggests that older women more commonly suffer from ill health than older men and that they are more likely to have multiple disabilities.
- Of particular concern in The Netherlands is the increased use of tranquilizers and barbiturates, especially among housewives and widows over age 40.
- Housing disadvantages are particularly likely to affect women because of their disproportionate representation among the very old and those living alone.
- Older women may therefore be more in need of care and support at older ages to enable them to maintain their independence. Yet they are more likely to have lost, through widowhood, one of their main sources of care (Coopmans *et al.*, 1989).

OTHER DANGER AREAS

There are, of course, many other areas of concern for older women which need detailed study. In the case of economy driven migration it is frequently the grandmother of the family who remains in the old homestead, sometimes charged with the total responsibility for small grandchildren, when the middle generation has virtually disappeared (Tout, 1989).

In another migratory phenomenon of modern days, the mass movements of refugees, there can be a sad and disastrous situation for older women in the matter of resettlement to a third country. Often it is only skilled or capable workers, with their spouses and children, who are resettled, leaving older women with least chance of impressing the resettlement selectors.

Another emergent distress signal is beginning to be heard from those areas where the strain of AIDS tends to favour a heterosexual route of transmission, in which case parts of eastern Africa appear to be greatly at risk. In such instances both spouses can be dying of AIDS, together possibly with one or two of the casually infected children. Because of the normal acceptance of a certain type of promiscuity and also of repeated marriages with younger wives, grandfather cohorts can also be infected or in any case will tend to predecease their female peers. This leaves the grandmother as the sole surviving adult able to fend for the infant family. Unfortunately it has to be said that, at the time of writing, the plight of that grandmother, as well as her heroic struggle to preserve the clan, do not attract the commitment of large funding sources which are preoccupied with biological and clinical priorities.

Other disadvantages of the older woman remain to be identified, researched and publicized. Some of them may be of little apparent statistical importance but can be of vital effect on the individual woman. An instance of this was discovered by a Bolivian agency when investigating the high incidence of eye problems in rural areas. It emerged that the women concerned had developed eye problems as a result of a lifetime of tending cooking fires in totally enclosed tiny houses, without windows or other ventilation, in a mountain zone with a frigid climate.

POSITIVE ACTION PROPOSED

Whilst most of the programmes, if not all, in this book will provide support for women, there are a number of actions and projects which already exercise positive discrimination, if not catering entirely for women. In fact, the use of day centres and clubs as referral and check points for health often 'favour' women who are the majority attenders as a rule. A Maltese project in this book refers to the difficulty of persuading males to attend such centres. A Belize study also noted this phenomenon to perhaps an even greater extent (Tout and Tout, 1985).

The Nairobi 'conversations' referred to earlier did not close on the note of apparent pessimism about elderly women's circumstances as might be inferred from quotations above. The conference went on to make some pertinent recommendations. Among these there were the following themes:

- To organize older women locally, regionally, nationally and internationally to promote their own economic and other interests.
- To ensure women's pension rights by valuing the domestic work which many women perform.
- To establish special income generating programmes for older women with initial input from governments or NGOs.
- To train older women to develop marketable skills so that they can obtain employment.
- To encourage women to buy goods and other services from other women and their specialized organisations.
- To use able younger-old women to support the more frail, especially where they are all living in some state of isolation.

A number of more general ageing conferences have also given some consideration to the special case of older women in their recommendations, advancing ideas such as:

- A special effort should be made to ensure that rural women of all ages are included and take an active part in the general course of development programmes.
- Legal provisions should be introduced so that, where this is not yet the case, widows have the right to full enjoyment of their deceased husbands' retirement benefits and rights.
- A return should be made to traditional, natural and simple styles of medicine and pharmacology in which older women were expert and which gave them a useful role in society.
- Older women should be used on a structured basis in work for which, at the moment, there may be a lack of workers, such as child minding, teaching assistants or in service industries, with additional credit imput to them for such time as they themselves may need care.
- To extol the achievements and prestige of those older women who have achieved notable deeds, in cultural events, politics, business or, increasingly, sport, as symbols for the mass media with a view to rectifying myths and stereotypes of the negative tendency (Tout, 1989).

POSITIVE ACTION TAKEN

Meanwhile, as gerontologists digest conference recommendations and national planners move through their sometimes prolonged processes, groups of older women have taken their destiny into their own hands in varying ways. The activities of larger groups are well known but a reference will be made here to a few lesser known initiatives. This may serve to conclude this brief commentary on a more optimistic note.

At the Nairobi conference already referred to, organisations cited as models included the Older Women's League, the Gray Panthers of the

USA and the Wise Elderly Women of The Netherlands. Of particular interest was the work of the International Friendship Circle located in Japan. This programme sponsors activities in Japan and shares the ideas with members from many other countries. One such project was the use of middle-aged and younger-old women, using their homemaking skills, in services such as the delivery of nutritious meals for older people unable to provide for themselves.

A similar operation in Peru provides meals for 120 elderly people daily. The providers of this service are a Grandparents Club which has unusual origins. Years ago a group of women gathered as pregnant and nursing mothers to discuss their mutual concerns as new mothers. They maintained their Mothers Club until they had graduated into grandmothers. At that stage they recognised that there were many of their peers who lived in great destitution and were suffering from stages of malnutrition. Their original talking club has now evolved into an action group which provides basic sustenance in a poverty stricken port area.

A similar initiative in the townships of South Africa succinctly sums up its services by changing the familiar title of Meals on Wheels to Meals on Foot. In another project, supported by HelpAge Kenya, the project title is more extended, but equally graphic as Women of Kichakasimba Take A Step Forward. As it implies, this is a self-help group of older women who are seeking and introducing ways of improving their entire community which, due to migration from the rural area, is heavily weighted to older people, with females in great majority. They have a poultry keeping project, a safe water scheme and other initiatives. An unusual aspect is the overnight guard duty undertaken by these older women to avoid losses from their valuable projects due to raiding thieves.

Programme planners have, however, been careful to avoid the kind of orientation of projects towards women which might develop into a segregation of older women. Whilst this may appear to be an extreme precaution there are sad instances of old people's homes, or sections of homes, which are exclusively devoted to women so that, at a particular point in a married couple's declining fortunes, they may have to suffer a kind of divorce in order that the woman may obtain the care she needs.

The reverse side of that coin is that the vast majority of programmes and activities which will improve the quality of life for elderly women are those which are non-segregated by sex, but which have some kind of insurance against any 'male chauvinistic' tendencies which may occur in the local culture.

LOOKING AHEAD

Perhaps the greatest immediate requirement is for governments and influential NGOs to add actions to their words and study, experiment, legislate, fund and implement fairly basic measures which would support the 'younger' woman carer upon whom the daily – and continuing for many years – responsibility falls for frontline support of an elder. Practical responses from authorities will range from respite provision through to national and local tax rebates, as well as actual cash grants and domiciliary resources support for the carer.

Whilst the traditional extended family (classically of three generations) tends to disintegrate, gerontologists are doomwatching on the increase of four and five generation families. Speculation may quite easily present cases where a great-grandmother, still able and alert, might have to be the carer for a less able and highly confused grandmother (Tout, 1989).

Speaking from a Canadian and North American perspective, Betty Havens (1991) says:

> It is startling that so little attention has been paid to the feminization of formal care ... in looking to the future of health care and aging with limited resources, it is imperative to know what women will do and how they will behave over the next several decades. There is little evidence from our Manitoba studies ... that consumption patterns will reverse, i.e. producing reductions in health service consumption by women ... we must also expect that women will continue to dominate as staff in the formal health system. We are less clear about whether they will continue to provide the requisite informal care, as more women work outside the home ...

From a European viewpoint, and surely with wider relevance, Sally Greengross (1991) says:

> The European Community and national governments will respond as older women begin to find their own voice ... The future of older women's issues at every level in Europe – local, regional, national and within the EC – depends partly on the ability of both lobbies, both the 'elderly' lobby and the 'women's' lobby, to take into consideration these important issues.

She concludes:

> Women's issues are an integral part of the challenge of an ageing population and should not be marginalized as society responds to this challenge.

Note: See also details on OWN, an older women's network, in Chapter 17.

The widow's predicament

43

Thoughts on a woman's role, especially the widow's, in a traditional society (India)

J.D. Pathak

Both socially and economically, women in India have been accorded a dependent and subservient position and their plight in old age has remained unheeded. Most of the older women in India are somehow, very often grudgingly, accommodated in families of their children.

Old age in women in India may be assumed to commence from the time of the menopause. On average, menopause in Indian women sets in at about the age of 45 years. By the age of 60 years, many women in India appear fairly aged. Most women of the well-to-do class lead a sedentary life. Their physical weakness is both a cause and effect of their inactivity.

India is a country of strong religious and social traditions. Historically they did not leave the old to their fate as obtained in some primitive savage societies. The status of women in India is even now, by and large, subsidiary to that of the man. Economic independence was denied to women. It seems that men, being the bread earners, could treat women as they liked.

THE TRADITIONAL ROLE

The *Manu Smriti*, a Hindu sacred writing, did not concede independent living to women: 'Woman is to be protected by father in childhood, by husband in youth, by sons in old age. A woman does not deserve independence!' Nevertheless, such an apparently harsh and unfair arrangement was not that harsh in its actual observation. In the family the woman had a more or less dignified and satisfying distribution of duties. 'The gods reside where women are respected', directed the same *Manu Smriti*.

The position of women in Islam was that of 'property' – property which could be disowned fairly easily. Yet normally Muslim women were not neglected in old age and they too lived with the families of sons or other relatives. The more progressive Parsee community permitted more independence and extended care of the old in a more organized way. The Christian society granted more economic as well as social freedom to women. Bombay is a cosmopolitan city wherein all citizens of all religions live their own way of life.

Mode of living modifies the life of human beings more than other factors. Active people live longer and healthier lives. Attitude to life is important. Worries precipitate senescence. So married people may live longer than unmarried or widowed, possibly because they are better looked after and are less likely to be drowned in their boredom, a common plight of the aged.

Over the years a woman's main role has been the family role and all the training given to a girl was aimed at enabling her to fill the roles of wife and mother. Her mother role continued for a long time in a joint family, only to be added to or replaced by the grandmother role. She retained these positions, however old, as long as the husband was alive.

Widowhood, however, generally brought about a change in the role. When the son or other heir becomes the head of the family, the daughter-in-law becomes the female head of the household and the old mother-in-law is relegated to a dependent role. Tension becomes inevitable unless the mother-in-law develops a positive attitude and the daughter-in-law is an understanding person.

Many an old woman is caught in the middle of two trends. She grew up in a culture which did not develop deep husband–wife relations because, in part, her spouse was still attached to his mother who ruled the household. Now in her old age she is faced with a modern daughter-in-law who is trying to replace her in her son's affections.

Childless widows have a harder time. They become dependent on other relatives, perhaps not so close in kinship and who have no real obligation. Often they become the family drudge. A widow is considered 'inauspicious' and is barred from some social events. Until the last century a widow was expected to commit *sati* (ritual suicide) or face ill treatment. Though *sati* has been abolished and the practice of it has stopped, ideas die hard and the restrictions remain – on diet, social contacts, physical appearance, etc. A widow without a child has no status at all in a family. She has no one she can relate to closely. She has nowhere else to go. Social stigma would be attached to any woman, however old, if she left the family home or the shelter afforded to her by her relations. Life for her can be dark and dismal.

Sister Subbalakshmi of Madras fought against this inhuman treatment of widows and established the Widows Home in Triplicane in Madras, where young widows were educated and taught crafts. Many of them are now old widows but are better able to cope for themselves.

CHANGING CIRCUMSTANCES

Conditions have changed tremendously today. Women have property rights by law, can adopt children and are allowed to remarry. But age-old, deep-rooted social stigmas prevent many from this solution. With increasing opportunities for education women are able to develop role flexibility and move into occupational careers, community service and other roles. But the lot of the poor, the illiterate and the uneducated aged woman is a cause for concern and calls for social action.

Older women also face another social problem. This is the conflict between the young and the old generations. The young consider the old as 'finished', that they have no more contribution to make, that their ideas in any case are outmoded. 'You don't understand', or 'You are too old to understand us' are common statements from the young.

The elderly women, especially those who have ruled their family, tend to be more orthodox in their outlook and are often critical of the young. A 'communication gap' develops between these two generations. While the elderly women cling desperately to their positions of authority, the young become militant and sometimes hostile. This situation causes a tension in the family circle and the older woman is unable to cope.

This tendency of clinging to power is also seen in other areas such as on committees, in politics, in self-employed positions. When family roles come to an end or occupational roles cease, they substitute leadership roles in organization or politics. The younger generation resents this continued occupation of leadership positions, while the older women are loath to give it up in favour of subsidiary or supportive roles.

Elderly women deserve better medical attention. Such care is not always easily available to them. The patients only come into hospital when they cannot get well at home under their own treatment. The plight of the old is often pitiable. They are frustrated. Very often their despondency stems from their traditional inferior economic and social status, from which they can imagine no exit. Though some economically well-off elderly women may have a satisfactory deal, the same is not true for all, particularly for the less fortunately placed.

In conclusion, changing structures and social order greatly affect women in old age. The older women of today are caught between two orders, the old with its rigid pattern of social relations and obligations and the new emerging order which is more flexible. There is also a new type of woman emerging who is educated and more independent and whose problems in her old age will be vastly different from those which women of former generations were subject to.

No adequate universal surveys or studies have yet been completed on the problems of women in old age or the problems of retired women. These did not constitute a serious problem of society until now, as they have been taken care of by the family. It is necessary to institute such studies and surveys to measure the depth and extent of the situation, so as to take necessary remedial measures to combat the present financial, health, housing and socio-economic problems, as well as to stay the tide of further escalation.

Note: Material drawn from a series of Bombay symposia organized by Dr Pathak with a significant contribution on widows by Kum E. Anchees of Bombay YWCA (Pathak, 1975).

PART FOURTEEN
Summing up

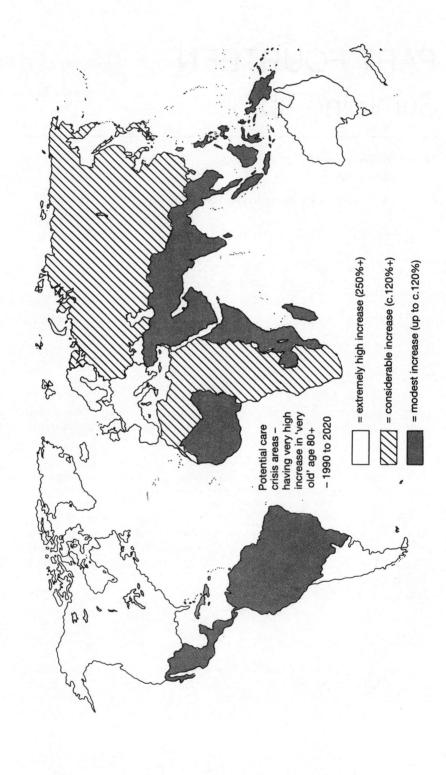

Potential care crisis areas – having very high increase in 'very old' age 80+ – 1990 to 2020

☐ = extremely high increase (250%+)

▨ = considerable increase (c.120%+)

▓ = modest increase (up to c.120%)

Reflections

44

Ken Tout

The great increase projected in the numbers of elderly people worldwide inevitably raises the question of how nations and local communities will cope with the accompanying increase in requirements for health and social services as well as direct financial support for older people or their families. The kind of prospect detailed by Alvarez at the beginning of this book suggests that some, if not all countries, will be gravely challenged at some point over the next 30 years to find the resources for adequate support to the elderly.

At the same time it is pointed out that decreasing fertility rates may mean that governments will be able to divert funds from one dependency group to another, so that the financial burdens resulting from increased numbers of elderly will be, to a certain extent, offset.

A recent authoritative United Nations publication takes a cautious view of this problem. Referring to studies which have already been made on the costs of future ageing programmes, it says:

> All of these studies indicate that public expenditure for the aged will increase as a result of population ageing. The studies also indicate, however, that these increases will be relatively modest when considered in the context of the economic growth expected to take place over the same period.
>
> *(Schulz, 1991)*

THE WARNING SIGNS

This concluding section will therefore resist the temptation to proclaim an economic catastrophe arising out of the rapid need to provide funds for health services for many more 'old old'; such services tend to cost up to seven times as much as those for younger cohorts. There is also the need for untold numbers of new pension and social security payments where at the moment few or none exist. It is necessary, therefore, to repeat some of the dangers pointed out earlier in this volume, such as:

- Eldemire's reference to the change in family composition, rising health costs and increased burdens on the community;
- Apt's warning that the well-being of the elderly has already become a 'crucial problem which requires urgent governmental action now';
- Bezrukov's note of the distancing of newly provided homes from the 'old haunts' of the elderly and consequent disruption of support systems;
- Pineda Soria's candid review of the inadequacy of existing services in a developed country, echoed by contributors from the USA and elsewhere.

Two further references might be introduced on this point. From a group of developing countries comes the comment as regards future cohorts of elderly:

> Unless these people are covered by an effective superannuation scheme, the burden of providing a taxation-based income support scheme for them may be too great for the shrinking population of working-age persons to bear. So although 2030 may seem a long way off, action is needed now...
>
> (Chen Ai Ju and Jones, 1989)

From a developed country another aspect is raised:

> The 'carers lobby' is becoming increasingly vocal as academics and others continue to quantify the financial implications of having caring responsibilities, for example, in terms of broken career paths, part-time work and increased expenditure.... How long governments will be able to ignore calls for an **adequate** carer's benefit to offset for such costs is debatable, but implicit central government reliance on unpaid family care as a means of controlling public expenditure may, and should be, short lived.
>
> (*Johnson and Falkingham, 1992*)

With these qualms in mind it becomes ever more necessary to examine the various options which are available in catering for a greying population. The types of programmes described briefly in this work need to be studied in more depth, evaluated, replicated and adapted as appropriate, but with a sense of urgency, even though 2030 may seem a long way off. For many older people an individual catastrophe has already struck in situations where there is as yet no sufficient preparation for the problem which has arisen.

It may be useful, therefore, to hark back to the question raised at the beginning of the book as to the usefulness of placing small key projects from developing countries alongside major developments in affluent societies. What are the commonalities, seeing that the diversities are so evident? What has each to say to each? And what have they in total to offer to the world?

LEARNING FROM EACH OTHER

In the introduction it was suggested that the luxurious elders' village in Florida, described by von Mering, had a basic principle to offer for ageing programmes at whatever level of economic development or in whatever culture they might be introduced. This was the principle of 'affinity bonding', the predetermining of a peaceful and happy group living experience by the careful selection of the groups which would live together. That the Florida group concerned was a 'WASP' one is irrelevant to the point. It is not too hard to imagine in most localities a situation where lack of affinity bonding might provoke violent repercussions among active elders forced to live together in some kind of irredeemable animosity.

Across the political spectrum, it is likely that some of Dacal's grandparents' houses and circles of elders in Cuba prosper more if there is cultural affinity between members. Others of the programmes described, such as in Cordoba, Argentina, reveal, by the diversity of activities offered, the inclination of older people to 'affinity bond' themselves together according to their own activity inclinations.

The present writer came across a variant of this principle, in its negative aspect, with regard to a lack of 'affinity' among families who consigned their relatives to old people's homes. A well-intentioned nun in Honduras had raised funds to construct a home which had two wings. The concept was that destitute elderly would live in one wing, whilst the other wing, totally detached, would be occupied by fee-paying elders from rich families. The fees would be sufficient to finance running costs for the two wings. In the event, the 'rich' wing remained almost empty. The families did not want their elders to be known to share an institution with destitute aged, even though physical contact would have been nil.

As also mentioned in introductory remarks, Kohli's point about appropriate provision is important as, referring to housing in particular, he says, 'Old people... are mainly not happy and do not feel at home in so-called "modern" surroundings, with a preponderance of glass and steel'. Leeson makes a similar point from a Danish point of view, taking into account availability of services, offering 'their own independent homes in contact with people... and in proximity of care and services as required and as individually assessed'. An overabundance of services may lead to loss of independence and self-motivation just as an excess of space or lavish furnishings may be unsettling to an older person of different tastes.

A very efficient order of sisters in Sucre, Bolivia, had been provided with an old military barracks which they had remodelled as an old people's home. Bedrooms had been tastefully furnished and had matching curtains and bedspreads. Care was beyond reproach. Yet the Mother Superior recorded a 50% drop-out of elderly peasants coming into the city home from the mountains. The room spaces were too large and the environment too sanitized, although care and food were excellent. The Mother Superior gave her opinion that the ideal old people's home for the rural elders would be a group of small, typical huts, where they could go on living in the traditional way, among their chickens and dogs, and maybe with a warden to watch over them.

The success of elderly pressure groups in industrialized societies means that now programmes are being introduced to meet the growing demand. As illustrated elsewhere, the rapidity of onset of ageing in a nation's population is likely to be considerably greater in developing countries in the future than it has been in industrialized societies in the past. New programmes are being introduced in those countries and some of them are described here.

ADEQUATE PREPARATION ESSENTIAL

However, in the rush to stop the gaps in services it is essential that adequate research and evaluation systems are invoked. Pineda Soria's integrated plan includes this element of prior investigation and assessment of need. My own experience in a decade of attempting to assist various developing country agencies with emergency welfare measures is that, to coin a phrase, 'We were often engaged in a fire brigade type of response when what we really needed was a squad of detectives'. Scarce resources can be wasted in a spate of sincere goodwill which aims at incorrect or even non-existent targets.

The evaluation process for pilot models is sometimes even more important than the prior investigation. Often data surfaces in the course of practical action where no data existed before. Sixsmith warns, with good reason, of the type of evaluation in which 'solutions to problems are already defined and evaluation amounts to little more than finetuning and rubber stamping'. Because of erroneous stereotypes about ageing and the inclination of good practitioners to impose their best treatment or service option upon elders seen as dependent, perhaps in no human field of evaluation are Sixsmith's two vital questions more necessary: 'Whose values dominate?' and 'In whose interests do services really operate?'.

In all supervisory processes of research, monitoring and evaluation it is important that the 'objects' of the process be incorporated realistically into the various activities so that they become human subjects and not units of data.

One writer, who has particularly examined the research processes in ageing, reports of the elders:

> Some have described the experience of 'being researched' as similarly disempowering to the experience of being on the receiving end of insensitive services... if researchers are asking for users to share with them often painful experiences, as well as give their time freely, they must be able to offer something in return.
>
> *(Barnes, 1992)*

Therefore, she continues, researchers:

> ...must find methods which maximise the possibility of change coming about as a result of the research, and of ensuring that those who are participants in the research process have access to and can use the results themselves.

Again those remarks apply equally to the various stages of monitoring and evaluation.

Turning to the family and home care, information from Rosenmayr and Boulasri, among others, points to a gradual breakdown of the traditional family everywhere. While methods will no doubt be sought to slow or reverse that breakdown, other methods will be needed to ensure adequate home care where the family is not able to offer all or any such care.

THE NEED FOR SENSITIVITY

Okada describes various levels of care support which can be put into a person's own home. However, there is some fear that local or national authorities may view home care as a cheaper alternative to other systems and may tend to evade the financial implications which still obtain in the best of home care. Johnson's remarks above reflect this fear. There is another danger, not so widely expressed, that the 'imposition' of home care may only serve to repeat some of the errors of institutionalization.

This area of concern has been studied by a researcher who says, 'Small wonder that the elderly have acquired the image of dependent, frail, needy, isolated people, for those are the "discreditable" facts most often recorded about them by home care services'. Referring to criticisms of institutions, the same writer continues:

> Home care for the frail and housebound does something very similar. It opens up the minutiae of personal life for examination and questioning by outsiders, strangers, authorities. The most simple and

previously taken-for-granted actions and needs have to be made public and humbly requested.

(Gavilan, 1992)

So home care, unthinkingly imposed or applied, is not an instant automatic panacea for all ills. And in the same vein, the bright prospects of aid held out by modern technology can only be of true solace to the elder if applied with sensitivity and restraint. The kind of robotic watcher described elsewhere might be seen by financial monitors as excusing cuts in staff ratios. It could also be psychologically disturbing to the unprepared sufferer from dementia who suddenly hears a disembodied voice retailing ghostly warnings.

There is no doubt that the Malta Good Neighbours Scheme is managed with extreme sensitivity because of its roots in what is virtually a more extended family structure. But both in the Malta programme and in the Pro Vida Colombia experience there is a further warning note about the limits to which volunteer support can be exercised. Garcia reports the need to supplement volunteers with qualified professionals or craftsmen as required. As with home care and the products of technology, volunteerism might be seen by financial monitors as another cheaper resource, but rarely can a volunteer group totally displace official and professional support.

Margolies and Achutti emphasize the need to bridge what has become known as the 'generation gap'. Various models have been introduced to counter misunderstandings between generations. Two similar programmes, one in the Volta region of Ghana and another in the most distant rural areas of Jamaica, use the strategy of sending school pupils to record memories of older people, ostensibly to be able to preserve records of traditional culture in national museums but with the very successful outcome of enhancing the intergenerational relationships.

Good residential practice permits access of younger generations to the resident elderly person. This is not a universal rule and the present writer has experience not only of young children being excluded from visiting opportunities but also of spouses being unable to have free contact. The enjoyment of residential life, for those who may need such provision, is usually enhanced by continued contact with the community. In some cases it has been possible, as McKenna and Jai Tout relate, for the central 'old people's home' function to become the hub of far wider community activity. As against this 'open door' policy the privacy of the resident must still be sacrosanct. There needs to be distinction between public and private places within an extended scheme.

The obvious remedy to the deficient areas which exist in some, or perhaps it should be **many**, residential establishments is an efficient council or committee of elders within the home. This might cause a few organizational dilemmas but, as Tunissen points out, the Gelderland experiments have been successful enough to warrant replication throughout The Netherlands.

Much depends on the sensitivities of the practitioner at all levels. Achutti and Gergely have indicated excellent measures to bridge that 'gap', in the one case by introducing students into an informal relationship with older patients and in the other by having the most eminent of specialists come to meetings of patients in order to have down-to-earth exchanges on all relevant subjects.

ELDERS EMPOWERED

Another 'gap', discernible even in the most highly structured of 'welfare states', is that between the formal and informal delivery systems. Reban proposes the Community Memory Project as one model of working towards interdisciplinary and multisectoral programmes. Leichsenring outlines counselling systems as a means of wedding formal and informal. But the latter makes the valid point that, in the urgency to wed authorities and disciplines, it is essential that 'the social competences of the elderly person and his/her carers gain an impact' and 'retain control over' any multi-authority contract.

The ability of elders to contribute conspicuously to the planning of their own destiny is stressed a number of times. Del Pozo and Ekongot supply evidence of considerable lateral thinking by elders in the evolution of useful projects. Chow and Kwan also refer to innovative activities, the former making a point with which many elderly might agree: 'the moral and cultural worth of the projects is regarded as being as important as, if not more important than, their economic value'. Again, the application of this principle can restrain the over-emphasis on economic imperatives which so often, and with good reason, become pre-eminent in programme planning.

Minkler's description of the Tenderloin project's strengthening of personal security and its impact on local crime is most reassuring in days when violence is proclaimed by the media to be of exceptional incidence. Research by the British Centre for Policy on Ageing tends to suggest that actual crime against older people is not as prevalent as is often supposed and is probably less than against other age groups. It is the fear of crime which impacts more on older persons and that fear is a real psychological experience which is as critical as actual bodily harm (Midwinter, 1990).

Empowerment of the elderly not only relates to security from danger in the broad light of day. It also concerns many more obscure and insalubrious aspects of life, ranging from elders' involvement in narcotic addiction to the reluctance of some medical professionals in a commercial medical system to treat elderly persons of uncertain resources. Indeed, Cox states categorically that one of the 'greatest barriers to expansion of the empowerment programme' had been the difficulty in 'convincing some more traditional practitioners that frail elderly can benefit from empowerment oriented approaches'.

Zaki and other have warned that the word 'empowerment', taken as a straight translation into some other languages, might be seen by the authorities of some countries to be politically unacceptable. This underlines one of the immediate problems of transfer of ideas and information cross-culturally. The writer attended a 1984 'expert group' meeting called by the United Nations to consider the possibility of standardization of terminologies (and methodologies) in gerontology. The general view at the time was pessimistic and subsequent progress has been slow, both in respect of direct literal translation of a term and of the comprehension of resulting concepts.

THE WEALTH OF ELDERLINESS

Fitness obviously enables the elder to pursue significant programmes of activity both in community service and in personal satisfaction. Esquivel presents a stimulating picture of activities within the AGECO programme with elders prominent in planning and organizing local groups. Bernard describes perhaps a somewhat more sophisticated structure but, in essence, not far removed from AGECO. The Peer Health Counsellor concept is as laudably illustrative of the best elements of elder action as the school pupils' health education presentations of Garcia's Pro Vida are of intergenerational action.

One factor too rarely discussed in some societies, but of paramount importance to the oldest persons, is the whole area of ultimate deterioration, dying, bereavement, the hereafter and burial. Some extended programmes, seeking to provide adequate services for all later stages of life, still separate the active living from the obviously dying. They hide the ultimate experience away in a manner in which the mentally ill and destitute elderly used to be hidden away. It is good to read of an environment like Queens Park Court where younger able residents can see through into the areas of living of the most frail and confused, still with their free choice systems, and know that there is a comfortable continuity in the days of their last ageing.

Both Mills and Machin present welcome insights into what have been sometimes considered darker corners of the human existence. There is wealth within dementia if the disturbing outer symptoms are discarded by the observer. There is no need to 'rage, rage' if suitable preparation, both of carers and care receivers, has gone before. At the same time it is to be wondered whether the so-called sophistication of modern life, in outlawing some of the traditional manifestations of grief, has led to a more sensible and sensitive attitude to death.

Here mention might be made of Hindu 'pre-death' houses. The simple homes of gurus, these are places where an old person can go to meditate and listen to wisdom and maybe to die quietly. Or, if death does not synchronize with that visit, to return home in a more tranquil and 'ready' state of mind. Another mention might be made of a Jamaican concept which derives from the British hospice system but which seeks to apply the hospice service on a domiciliary basis with the minimum of 'in' beds available only for the most extreme circumstances.

Nyanguru and McKenna both recognize the importance of the after-death arrangements. For years the elderly nun ran a simple funeral programme in Beni, herself making coffins when there was no other alternative, in order to give reassurance to dying elders to whom the burial was of supreme importance. Nyanguru in his description of Melfort develops the theme of concern of southern Africans. Even in the UK Age Concern and Help the Aged have been drawn into action to provide an insured area of solace and peace for which Welfare State provisions are not – and perhaps never could be – totally adequate.

TRANSNATIONAL TRANSFERS

One aspect which has not received specific treatment in this volume has, however, been referred to in the course of several reviews and is implicit in almost all sections of the work. This is the question of transfer of resources. Often such 'aid' is seen as representing an export from more 'advanced' countries to the developing world. But, as Reban says, 'nor must the transfer of experience be always in one direction' for even among the gerontologically advanced nations 'none would yet claim to have devised a model which is comprehensive, widely available and generally affordable' (either by the state or the individual person).

It is to be hoped that this study provides ideas and information which will further stimulate the trend towards a true cross-cultural, multilateral exchange of ideas, based on the acknowledgement of the many commonalities in ageing worldwide, as well as the value of the diversities.

What concerns the present writer is that the increase in interest in cross-cultural conferences on ageing and the proliferation of resolutions and recommendations seem to be galloping ahead of political will in some instances and, more generally, of serious application to the question of international aid. Whilst the developing countries can feed excellent concepts and project experience into the international pool of resources, any considerable transfer in cash and materials – as well as some skills – needs to be on a North to South basis, parallel to the existing routeings of international development aid.

Whilst nations of the world subscribed to the recommendation of the World Assembly on Ageing in 1982 and ratified the setting up of a United Nations Trust Fund on Ageing, there has been a reluctance on the part of a number of nations to include the subject of ageing in major developmental aid transfers. It has been argued (to the writer by officials of governmental aid departments) that aid to elders is 'down the drain' welfare expenditure and that elderly programmes cannot be seen as developmental because old people do not live long enough.

Such arguments are simplistic in the extreme and do no credit to those who propound them. Any measure which lightens the future national and local burden of expenditure on increasing care services for the elderly must be seen as developmentally beneficial to the country concerned. Any programme which pumps new wealth into a starved economy, at whatever community level, must be acknowledged as a unit of development. There are examples enough in this book of such programmes and many more which could be mentioned.

In recent years the European Community has acknowledged that 'ageing' should be listed as an appropriate subject for its CEC DGVIII aid to developing countries fund. One example of this co-funding co-operation was substantial assistance to enable the implementation of a national plan on ageing in Belize (as set out in Tout and Tout, 1985). Also the Vilcabamba, Ecuador, and Zabbaleen, Egypt, projects attracted CEC support. The Canadian Government, through its CIDA system, has also been generous, with Pro Vida Colombia and other similar systems as beneficiaries. Other national governments have also made co-funding contributions (that is, making an aid grant equivalent to a non-governmental input for the same project).

Having said that, the total of actual financial transfer, either directly to the United Nations Trust Fund or by co-funding through NGOs, since the World Assembly on Ageing has been miniscule compared with spending on non-humanitarian programmes, or even with the vast amounts of aid diverted to victims of major disaster emergencies.

This is obviously a subject for long and detailed debate but it might be permissible here to make one proposal. The vision of a potential ageing crisis was accepted as justifiable at the 1982 Assembly. On 15 and 16 October 1992 the United Nations General Assembly returned to the issue, without significant dissentient voices or votes against proposals in which Julia Alvarez was a prime mover. (Schulz, 1991, and Tout, 1992, contributed to the recent debate.)

If, therefore, the nations of the world accept the possibility that over the next three decades the ageing of the population may constitute a considerable socio-economic crisis unless suitable action is taken in the meantime, why not act as follows?

There already exists a United Nations accord by which wealthier member states pledge to work towards allocating aid equivalent to 0.7% of the gross national product to stimulate world development. In general that target has not been reached. Some nations are still working around a percentage only halfway to the target. But even 0.35% of the GNP of a major nation is a great amount of finance available for transfer. The problem lies in the allocation of such transfers.

Given the United Nations consensus on the importance of the ageing issue and given the general recognition that developing countries will age more rapidly with significant problems for weaker economies, let the donor countries deliberately allocate an agreed amount of their aid to ageing. Let that aid equal a percentage of their current GNP allocation equal to the current average percentage of elderly in the population of developing countries. That would mean, say, that about 5% of a country's present 0.35% (or whatever level) of GNP allocation to overseas aid would go to ageing programmes.

This would be a considerably higher contribution than at present and could be channelled in many ways (to the Trust Fund, the new Banyan Fund, co-funding to NGOs or bilaterally between nations) and could consist of cash, materials, skills, information and other requisite resources.

A CALL TO ACTION

Above all, this book would achieve a prime aim if it became a call to action. There are sufficient examples in this study to show that academics and researchers can link hands with programme planners, carers and care receivers so that good principles, innovative ideas and illuminating research are translated quickly into action.

An introductory note was provided by Ambassador Julia Alvarez who, not satisfied with debating and lobbying the world's governments, was a prime mover in the establishment of the Banyan Fund as an independent fundraising instrument with full support of the United Nations. The other introductory note was from Nana Apt who is a busy teacher and researcher, but finds time to launch a PanAfrican debate and to assist in the setting up of the HelpAge Ghana movement.

Optimism is also engendered by the thought of the many busy gerontologists who freely gave time to contribute to this book, in spite of impending deadlines of their own, because of their belief in the need for cross-cultural debate and action on ageing in the immediate future.

Much has been said about the active participation of older people in such debate. And in case anyone should be tempted to ask the wily question, 'Where is the voice of the senior, the retiree, the elder, in this book?' it might be pertinent now to reply, 'There are Alvarez, Garcia, Kohli, McKenna, Pathak, von Mering, Zaki and Tout, K., at least', not to stretch the definitions too far!

A concept for ageing to the year 2001

On 15 and 16 October 1992 the United Nations General Assembly debated the issue of world ageing, thus marking the ten year period since the World Assembly on Ageing of 1982. In preparation for the 1992 debate a group of experts was invited to consider proposing targets at both global and national levels for the next decade to the year 2001.

Ken Tout was asked to prepare a preliminary background paper on these issues. In order to express the basic principles of ageing programmes in a concise and easily comprehensible style he evolved the acronym 'DESIR' as set out below.

DIGNITY	preserving/restoring older persons' dignity
EDUCATION	through education of elders/carers/public/nation
SUPPORT	leading to family and community support assurance
INDEPENDENCE	encouraging independence achieved or enhanced by rehabilitation
REHABILITATION	in physical, mental and socio-economic condition

Not imposing upon the elder alien and dependency making regimes, but enabling each person to generate his/her own best lifestyle, with appropriate support.

The French *desir* = desire, aim, aspiration

(*Tout, 1992*)

References

Abraham, D. (1989) Reaching elderly abandoned citizens housebound, in *Aging, Demography and Well-being in Latin America*, (eds M.D. Alvarez, O. von Mering and K. Tout), Center for Gerontological Studies, University of Florida, Gainesville, Florida, pp. 87–92.

Ageing International (1989) **XVI**(2), 13 (Norwegian experiments in breaking down dichotomy between community and nursing home care).

Andrews, G., Esterman, E.J., Braunack-Mayer, A.J. and Rungie, C.M. (eds) (1986) *Aging in the Western Pacific*, WHO Regional Office, Manila.

Aponte Bolivar, M. (1978) *El Anciano en la Sociedad Venezolana*, Universidad Central de Venezuela, Caracas.

Apt, N.A. (1971) *Socio-economic Conditions of the Aged in Ghana*, Department of Social Welfare and Community Development monograph, Accra.

Apt, N.A. (1989) *Impact and Consequences of Social Change on Aging in Ghana*, Sociology Department, University of Ghana, Legon.

Apt, N.A. (1991) Ghanaian youth on aging: a survey report. *BOLD*, **1**(3), 18–21.

Attias-Donfut, C. and Rosenmayr, L. (eds) (1993) *Vieillir en Afrique*, Presses Universitaires, Paris.

Ball, C. (1992) Promoting productive, creative and independent ageing: the experience of FAIAF in Argentina. *Community Development Journal* **27**(2), 140–8.

Barnes, M. (1992) Beyond satisfaction surveys: involving people in research. *Generations Review*, **2**(4), 15–17.

Berger, P. and Neuhaus, R. (1977) *To Empower People*, American Enterprise Institute, Washington DC.

Bernard, M. and Ivers, V. (1986) Peer Health Counselling: a way of countering dependency?, in *Dependency and Interdependency in Old Age: Theoretical Perspectives and Policy Alternatives* (eds C. Phillipson, M. Bernard and P. Strang), Croom Helm, London.

Bernard, N. and Phillipson, C. (1991) Self-care and health in old age, in *Nursing Elderly People*, 2nd edn., (ed. S.J. Redfern), Churchill Livingstone, Edinburgh.

Bezrukov, V.V., Gichev, Y.P., Chaikovskaya, V.V., Sidorov, A.I. and Povorosniuk, V.V. (1991) Automated system for quantitative assessment of risk to lose self-care abilities as a new approach to defining needs of the elderly in various kinds of medical and social services. *Problemy Starenia i Dolgoletia* (Problems of Ageing and Longevity), **1**(1), 63–9 (in Russian).

Bocian, K. and Newman, S. (1989) Evaluation of intergenerational programs: why and how?, in *Intergenerational Programs*, (eds S. Newman and S.W.

Brummel), Haworth, New York.

Brodaty, H. and Peters, K.E. (1992) Cost effectiveness of a training program for dementia carers. *International Psychogeriatrics*, **4**(1), 11–22.

Chen Ai Ju and Jones, G. (1989) *Ageing in ASEAN: Its Socio-economic Consequences*, Institute of Southeast Asian Studies, Singapore.

Chow, N.W.S. (1987) Western and Chinese ideas of welfare. *International Social Work*, **30**, 31–41.

Chow, N.W.S. (1991) Does filial piety exist under Chinese communism? *Journal of Aging and Social Policy*, **3**(1/2), 209–25.

Conable, C.W. (1986) *Conversations in Nairobi: Aging and the Global Agenda for Women*, American Association for International Aging, Washington DC.

Consumer Reports (1991 and 1992) US Government Printing Office, Washington DC.

Cook, T.D. and Shadish, W.R. (1986) Program evaluation: the worldly science. *Annual Review of Psychology*, **37**, 193–232.

Coopmans, M., Harrop, A. and Hermans-Huiskes, M. (1989) *The Social and Economic Situation of Older Women in Europe*, Commission of the European Communities, Brussels.

Cox, E.O. (1988) Empowerment of low-income elderly in group work. *Social Work with Groups*, **11**(4), 111–25.

Cox, E.O. (1991) The critical role of social action in empowerment-oriented groups, in *Action in Group Work* (eds A. Vinik and M. Levin), Haworth, New York.

Cronbach, L.J. (1986) Social inquiry by and for earthlings, in *Metatheory in Social Science* (eds D.W. Fiske and R.A. Shweder), University of Chicago Press, Chicago.

Davis-Friedmann, D. (1991) *Long Lives: Chinese Elderly and the Communist Revolution*, Stanford University Press, Stanford.

Dryzek, J. (1982) Policy analysis as a hermeneutic activity. *Policy Sciences*, **14**, 309–29.

Engelhardt, K.G. (1989) Health and human service robotics: multidimensional perspectives. *International Journal of Technology and Aging*, **2**(1), 6–41.

Fernandez-Pereiro, A. and Sanchez-Ayendez, M. (1992) LinkAges: building bridges between children and the elderly. *Ageing International*, **19**(2), 10–14.

Finansy I Statistika (1990) (in Russian – Demographic Yearbook), USSR Government Office, Moscow.

Fortes, M. (1984) Age, generation and social structure, in *Age and Anthropological Theory* (eds D.I. Kertzer and J. Keith), Cornell University Press, Ithaca

Garrett, M. (1992) *Ageing in the Developing World: Trends and Needs*, International Institute on Ageing, Malta (unpublished).

Gavilan, H. (1992) Care in the community: issues of dependency and control – the similarities between institution and home. *Generations Review*, **2**(4), 9–12.

Gibran, K. (1972) *The Prophet*, Heinemann, London.

Gibson, M.J. (1985) *Older Women around the World*, International Federation on Aging, Washington DC.

Gilster, S.D. and McCracken, A.L. (1991) A unique teaching opportunity: a specialized facility for persons with Alzheimer's disease. *Educational Gerontology*, **17**(6), 621–30.

Gitlin, L.N. and Corcoran, M. (1991) Training occupational therapists in the care of the elderly with dementia and their caregivers: focus on collaboration. *Educational Gerontology*, **17**(6), 591–606.

Glendenning, F. (ed.) (1985) *New Initiatives in Self-Health Care for Older People*, The Beth Johnson Foundation, Stoke-on-Trent.

Glendenning, F. (ed.) (1986) *Working Together for Health: Older People and Their Carers*, The Beth Johnson Foundation, Stoke-on-Trent.

Greengross, S. (1991) Women's issues in an ageing society. *BOLD*, **2**(1), 12–14.

Gutierrez, L.M. (1990) Working with women of color; an empowerment perspective. *Social Work*, **March**, 149–52.

Hampson, J. (1982) *Old Age: A Study of Ageing in Zimbabwe*, Mambo, Gweru.

Hanley, I. and Hodge, J. (1984) *Psychological Approaches to the Care of the Elderly*, Methuen, London.

Harootyan, R.A. (1991) A brave new world of ageing in the 21st century. *Ageing International*, **18**(1), 22–4.

Havens, B. (1991) Interface of the formal system and informal care. *BOLD* **2**(1), 15–17.

Hopson, B. and Scally, M. (1981) *Lifeskills Teaching*, McGraw Hill, London.

Ivers, V. and Meade, K. (1991) *Older Volunteers and Peer Health Counselling: A New Approach to Training and Development*. The Beth Johnson Foundation, Stoke-on-Trent.

Johansson, L. (1990) Group dwellings for dementia patients. *Ageing International*, **16**(1), 34–7.

Johnson, P. and Falkingham, J. (1992) *Ageing and Economic Welfare*, Sage, London.

Kane, R. Evans, J.G. and Macfadyen, D. (eds) (1990) *Improving the Health of Older People: A World View*, Oxford University Press, Oxford.

Kendig, H., Hashimoto, A. and Coppard, L.C. (eds) (1992) *Family Support for the Elderly: The International Experience*, Oxford Medical Publications, Oxford.

Kinsella, K.G. (1988) *Aging in the Third World*, Center for International Research, US Bureau of the Census, Washington, DC.

Kosberg, J. (ed.) (1992) *Family Care of the Elderly: Social and Cultural Changes*, Sage, Newbury Park.

Kosberg, J. and Tobin, S. (1972) Variability among nursing homes. *The Gerontologist*, **12**, 214–19.

Kubler-Ross, E. (1973) *On Death and Dying*, Tavistock, London.

Kwan, A.Y.H. (1991) *A Study of the Coping Behaviour of Caregivers in Hong Kong*, Writers' and Publishers' Co-operative, Hong Kong.

Lincoln, Y.S. and Guba, E.G. (1985) *Naturalistic Enquiry*, Sage, Beverly Hills.

Littlewood, J. (1990) *Aspects of Grief*, Routledge & Kegan Paul, London.

MAAS (1985) *Les Personnes Agées au Maroc*, Ministère de l'Artisanat et des Affaires Sociales, Rabat, Morocco.

Machin, L. (1990) *Looking at Loss*, Longman, London.

Margolies, L. (1990) *Issues of Cross-cultural Transferability of Model Programs for the Aged*, International Exchange Center on Gerontology, University of South Florida, Tampa.

Mazzei Berti, J.E. (1988) *La Mejor Edad*, Italgrafica, Caracas.

McCallum, J. and Howe, A.L. (1992) Family care of the elderly in Australia, in *Family Care of the Elderly*, (ed. J. Kosberg), Sage, Newbury Park.

McLaughlin, M.W. (1985) Implementation realities and evaluation design, in *Social Science and Social Policy* (eds R.L. Shotland and M.M. Mark), Sage, Beverly Hills.

Midwinter, E. (1990) *The Old Order: Crime and Older People*, Centre for Policy on Ageing, London.

Miesen, B.M.L. (1990) *Gehechtheid en Dementie*, University of Nijmegen, Nijmegen.

Mills, M. (1991) *Making the Invisible Visible. A Qualitative Study in the Use of Reminiscence Therapy and Counselling Skills with Dementing Elderly People*, Bournemouth Polytechnic, Bournemouth.

Ministry of Health and Welfare (1991) *National Health Statistics*, Ministry of Health and Welfare, Tokyo, Japan.

Moore, J. (1992) New potential looms among affinity groups: classic concept drives novel strategies. *Contemporary Long Term Care*, **15**(6), 26–101.

Muchena, O. (1978) *African Aged in Towns*, Harare School of Social Work, Harare.

Nusberg, C. (1990) Job training for older workers lags in the industrialized world. *Ageing International*, **16**(1), 23–30.

Nyanguru, A. (1985) *Residential Care for the Black Destitute Elderly*, Harare School of Social Work, Harare.

Nyanguru, A. (1987) Residential care for the destitute elderly, *Journal of Cross-cultural Gerontology*, 2, 345–57.

Nyanguru, A. (1990) The quality of life of the elderly living in institutions and homes for the elderly. *Journal for Social Development in Africa*, 5(2), 25–43.

Nyanguru, A. and Peil, M. (1991) *Zimbabwe since independence, a people's assessment. African Affairs*, **90**, 607–20.

Onyx, J., Benton, P. and Bradfield, J. (1992) Aged services in Australia – community development and government response. *Community Development Journal*, **27**(2), 166–74.

Oswald, W.D. and Gunzelmann, T. (1992) Functional rating scales and psychometric assessment in Alzheimer's disease. *International Psychogeriatrics*, **4**(Supplement 1), 79–88.

Parsons, R.J. (1991) Empowerment as a principle and product in social work practice. *Social Work with Groups*, **11**(3/4), 31–45.

Pathak, J.D. (1975 and subsequent) *A Symposium on Problems of Women in Old Age*, Bombay Medical Research Centre, Bombay.

Prime Minister's Office (1981) *Survey of Japanese Elderly*, Prime Minister's Office, Tokyo, Japan.

Rangel, L.E. (1988) Elderly councils in Mexico. *Danish Medical Bulletin*, Special Supplement Series No. 6.

Riker, H.C. (1990) Living is a continuing process, in *Retirement Counselling: A Practical Guide*, (eds H.C. Riker and J.E. Myers), Hemisphere, New York.

Rivlin, A.M. and Wiener, J.M. (1988) *Caring for the Disabled Elderly: Who will Pay?* Brookings Institution, Washington DC.

Rosenman, L.S. and Winocur, S. (1990) Australian women and income security for old age: a cohort study. *Journal of Cross-cultural Gerontology*, 5(3), 277–91.

Rosenmayr, L. (1991) Improving the health status of the rural elderly in Mali. *Journal of Cross-cultural Gerontology* 6(3), 301–18.

Rosenmayr, L. (1992) *Die Schnüre vom Himmel*, Böhlau, Vienna.

Rossi, P.H., Freeman, H.E. and Wright, S.R. (1979) *Evaluation: A Systematic Approach*, Sage, Beverly Hills.

Russell, B. (1976) *Mysticism and Logic*, Allen and Unwin, London.

Schulz, J. (1991) *The World Ageing Situation 1991*, United Nations, New York.

Sixsmith, A.J. (1993) *Frameworks for Understanding Quality of Life*, Open University Press, Milton Keynes.

Somers, A.R. and Spears, N.L. (1992) *The Continuum Care Retirement Community: A Significant Option for Long-term Care?*, Springer, New York.

Sweeting, H. (1991) Caring for a relative with dementia: anticipatory grief and social death. *Generations*, **16**, 6–11.

Tilson, D. (1990) *Aging in Place: Supporting the Frail Elderly in Residential Environments*, Scott, Foresman, Glenview, Il.

Tout, K. (1989) *Ageing in Developing Countries*, Oxford University Press, Oxford.

Tout, K. (1992) *Ageing: Programme Recommendations at the National Level for the Year 2001*, United Nations CSDHA, Vienna.

Tout, K. and Tout, J. (1985) *Perspectives on Ageing in Belize*, HelpAge International/OPEC, London.

von Mering, O. (1992a) Societies in transition: the impact of longevity on generations, *Educational Gerontology*, **18**, 123–34.

von Mering, O. (1992b) *Beyond the Concept of Successful Aging: A Transcultural and Individual Perspective*, Southern Regional Education Board Press, Atlanta, Ga.

Weick, K.E. (1984) Small wins: redefining the scale of social problems. *American Psychologist*, **39**, 40–9.

Wilson, G. (1991) Models of ageing and their relation to policy formation and service provision. *Policy and Politics*, **19**(1), 37–47.

Worden, W. (1990) *Grief Counselling and Grief Therapy*, Tavistock, London.

Further reading

Alvarez, M.D., von Mering, O. and Tout, K. (1989) *Aging, Demography and Well-being in Latin America*, Center for Gerontological Studies, University of Florida, Gainesville, Florida.

Bengtson, V.L. and Schaie, K.W. (eds) (1989) *The Course for Later Life: Research and Reflections*. Springer, New York.

Binstock, R.H. and George, L.K. (eds) (1990) *Aging and the Social Sciences*, Academic Press, New York.

Blaikie, A. (1992) Whither the third age? Implications for gerontology. *Generations Review*, **2**(1), 2–4.

Bold (1991), 2 (1). Special issue on elderly and aging women.

Bond, J. and Coleman, P. (eds) (1990) *Ageing in Society: An Introduction to Social Gerontology*, Sage, London.

Brubaker, E. (1987) *Working with the Elderly: A Social Systems Approach*, Sage, Newbury Park.

Butler, R.N. and Bearn, A.G. (eds) (1985) *The Aging Process, Therapeutic Implications*, Raven Press, New York.

Cowgill, D.O. (1986) *Aging Around the World*, Wadsworth, Belmont, Ca.

Coyle, J.M. (1991) *Families and Aging: A Selected Annotated Bibliography*, Greenwood Press, Connecticut.

Crosby, G. (ed) (1991) *Old Age: A Register of Social Research 1985–90*, Centre for Policy on Ageing, London.

Cunningham, W.R. (1989) Intellectual abilities and age, in *The Course for Later Life: Research and Reflections* (eds V.L. Bengtson and K.W. Schaie), Springer, New York.

Danish Medical Bulletin, Special Supplement Series No. 6, 1988 *Community-based initiatives to reduce social isolation and to improve health of the elderly*.

Decalmer, P. and Glendenning F. (1993) *The Abuse and Mistreatment of Elderly People*, Sage, London.

Denham, M.J. (1990) *Care of the Long Stay Elderly Patient*, Chapman & Hall, London.

Di Gregorio, S. (1987) *Social Gerontology: New Directions*, Croom Helm, Beckenham.

Dickinson, D. and Johnson, M. (eds) (1992) *Death, Dying and Bereavement*, Sage, London.

Evandrou, M. (1987) *The Use of Domiciliary Services by the Elderly: A Survey*, London School of Economics, London.

Evers, A. and Svetlik, I. (eds) (1991) *New Welfare Mixes in Care for the Elderly*, Volume 1, Eurosocial Report 40/1, European Centre, Vienna.

Feil, N. (1992) *VALIDATION: The Feil Method: How to Help Disoriented Old-Old*, Edward Feil Productions, Cleveland, Ohio.

Fennell, G., Evers, H. and Phillipson, C. (1988) *The Sociology of Old Age*, Open University Press, Milton Keynes.

Finch, J. (1989) *Family Obligations and Social Change*, Basil Blackwell, Oxford.

Francis, S.E. (1988) *Programmes and Projects for the Elderly in the Caribbean Which Combat Loneliness and Isolation*, University of West Indies, Kingston, Jamaica.

Garrett, G. and Payne, K. (eds) (1992) *Adding Health to Years*, HelpAge International, London.

Garrod, G. (1993) The mistreatment of elderly people – where to now?

BASELINE, Journal of the British Association for Service to the Elderly, **51**, 27–40.

Gibson, H.B. (1991) *The Emotional and Sexual Lives of Older People*, Chapman & Hall, London.

Glasse, L. and Hendricks, J. (eds) (1991) *Gender and Aging*, Baywood, Amityville, NY.

Hayslip, B. jun. and Leon, J. (1992) *Hospice Care*, Sage, Newbury Park.

INIA (International Institute on Aging) (1990) *Short-term Training in Income Security for the Elderly in Developing Countries*, INIA/United Nations, Malta.

Jeffries, M. (ed.) (1989) *Growing Old in the Twentieth Century*, Routledge & Kegan Paul, London.

Jones, G.M.M. and Miesen, B.M.L. (eds) (1992) *Care Giving in Dementia: Research and Applications*, Tavistock/Routledge, London.

Kendig, H.L. (1986) *Ageing and Families*, Allen and Unwin, Australia.

Kinsella, K.G. (1990) *Living Arrangements of the Elderly and Social Policy: A Cross-national Perspective*. US Bureau of the Census, Washington DC.

Kosberg, J.I. (1993) *International Handbook on Community Services for the Elderly*, Greenwood, Westport, CT.

Kosberg, J.I. and Garcia, O.L. (1991) Social changes affecting family care of the elderly. *Journal of the International Institute on Aging*, **1**(2), 2–5.

Laczko, F. and Victor, C.R. (eds) (1992) *Social Policy and Older People*, Avebury, Aldershot.

Lawton, M.P. and Herzog, A.R. (eds) (1992) *Special Research Methods for Gerontology*, Baywood, Amityville, NY.

Marshall, M. (1991) *Working with Dementia: Guidelines for Professionals*, Venture, Birmingham.

Martin, L.G. (1991) Population aging policies in East Asia and the United States. *Science*, **251**, 527–31.

McClymont, M., Thomas, S. and Denham, M.J. (1991) *Health Visiting and Elderly People: A Health Promotion Challenge*, Churchill Livingstone, Edinburgh.

McEwen, E. (ed.) (1990) *Age: The Unrecognised Discrimination*, ACE/Age Concern England, London.

Meredith, B. (1993) *The Community Care Handbook*, ACE/Age Concern England, London.

Minkler, M. and Estes, C. (eds) (1991) *Critical Perspectives on Aging: The Political and Moral Economy of Growing Old*, Baywood, Amityville, NY.

Monk, A. and Cox, C. (1991) *Home Care for the Elderly: An International Perspective*, Auburn House, New York.

Morgan, K. (ed.) (1992) *Gerontology: Responding to an Ageing Society*, Jessica Kingsley, London.

Myers, G.C. (1990) Demography of aging, in *Handbook of Aging and The Social Sciences* (eds R.H. Binstock and L.K. George), Academic Press, New York.

Neill, J. and Williams, J. (1992) *Leaving Hospital: A Study of Elderly People and their Discharge to Community Care*, HMSO for NISW, London.

Neugarten, B. (1986) *Middle Age and Aging*, University of Chicago Press, Chicago.

Newman, S. and Brummel, S.W. (1989) *Intergenerational Programs: Imperatives, Strategies, Impacts, Trends*, Haworth, New York.

Nusberg, C. and Sokolovsky, J. (1990) *The International Directory of Research and Researchers in Comparative Gerontology*, IFA, Washington DC.

Osgood, N.J., Brant, B.A. and Lipman, A. (1991) *Suicide Among the Elderly in Long-term Facilities*, Greenwood, New York.

Peace, S.M. (ed.) (1990) *Researching Social Gerontology: Concepts, Methods and Issues*, Sage, London.

Phillipson, C. and Biggs, S. (1992) *Understanding Elder Abuse: A Training Manual for Helping Professionals*, Longman, London.

Plett, P.C. and Lester, B. (1991) *Training for Older People – A Handbook*. International Labour Office, Geneva.

Pritchard, J. (1992) *The Abuse of Elderly People*, Jessica Kingsley, London.

Robertson, S.E. and Brown, R.I. (eds) (1992) *Rehabilitation Counselling: Approaches in the Field of Disability*, Chapman & Hall, London.

Rosenmayr, L. (1986) *More than Wisdom: Research and Reflection on the Position of Old Age in Traditional and Changing African Society*, University of Vienna, Vienna.

San Diego State University (1993) *Population Aging: International Perspectives*. Proceedings from the International Conference on Population Aging held in San Diego, CA, September 1992.

Schmahl, W. (ed.) (1989) *Redefining the Process of Retirement: An International Perspective*, Springer, New York.

Schulz, J., Borowski, A. and Crown, W.H. *Economics of Population Aging: The 'Graying' of Australia, Japan and the United States*, Greenwood, Connecticut.

Sheppard, H.L. and Streib, G. (1985) *Aging in China*, International Exchange Center on Gerontology, Tampa.

Sokolovsky, J. (1986) *Growing Old in Different Societies: Cross-cultural Perspectives*, Coply Publishing, Acton, Mass.

Streib, G.F. (1987) Retirement communities, in *The Encyclopedia of Aging*, (ed. G.L. Maddox), Springer, New York.

Tout, K. (1985) The community against ageing problems in the third world. *COMM* (European Clearing House for Community Work), **26**, 252–61.

Tout, K. (1988) Aging: social supports for the elderly and community interventions in developing countries. *Danish Medical Bulletin*, Special Supplement, No. 6, 67–72.

Tout, K. (1989) Intergenerational exchange in developing countries, in *Intergenerational Programs: Imperatives, Strategies, Impacts, Trends* (eds) S. Newman and S.W. Brummel, Haworth, New York.

Tout, K. (1992a) Debt, duty and demands in third world ageing: the role of education. *Journal of Educational Gerontology*, **7**(1), 25–35.

Tout, K. (1992b) Does third age plus third world equal third class? *Community Development Journal*, **27**(2), 122–9.

Tout K. (1992c) A more distant age. *Generations Review*, **2**(2), 9–12.

Tout, K. (1993) Empowerment: an aging perspective, in *Population Aging: International Perspectives*, San Diego State University.

United Nations Department of International Economic and Social Affairs (UNDIESA) (1991) *World Population Prospects 1990*. ST/ESA/SER.A/120, New York.

Victor, C. (1991) *Health and Health Care in Later Life*, Open University Press, Milton Keynes.

Walker, A., Guillemard, A.-M. and Alber, J. (eds) (1991) *Social and Economic Policies and Older People*, First Annual Report of the European Community Observatory, CEC, Brussels.

Walker, J. (1991) *Preparing for Retirement: the Employer's Guide*, Age Concern England/Pre-Retirement Association of Great Britain and Northern Ireland, London.

Warnes, A.M. (1989) *Human Ageing and Later Life: Multidisciplinary Perspectives*, Edward Arnold, London.

Wilcocks, D., Peace, S. and Kellaher, L. (1987) *Private Lives in Public Places: A Research-based Critique of Residential Life in Local Authority Old People's Homes*, Tavistock, London.

Williams, E.I. (1989), *Caring for Elderly People in the Community*, Chapman & Hall, London.

Worsley, J. (1990) *Taking Good Care: A Handbook for Care Assistants*, ACE/Age Concern England, London.

Worsley, J. (1992) *Good Care Management: A Guide to Setting Up and Managing a Residential Home*, ACE/Age Concern England, London.

Wright, S.G. (1988) *Nursing the Older Patient*, Chapman & Hall, London.

Yang, Z. and Xu, Y. (eds) (1990) Strategic research on aging problems in Shanghai, in *Life Style of the Elderly in Villages and Cities*, Shanghai Municipal Aging Committee and Shanghai Society for Gerontology, Shanghai.

Index